THE
WHITE GAME

ACHIEVING PEAK PERFORMANCE
WITH THE POWER OF PRESENCE

**PETER KRONIG &
CHRIS CORBETT**

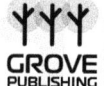

GROVE
PUBLISHING

© Peter Kronig and Chris Corbett 2021

All rights reserved. No part of this publication may be reproduced, stored in a retrieval system, or transmitted in any form or by any means electronic, mechanical, photocopying, recording, or otherwise, without the prior permission of both the copyright owner and the above publisher of this book.

ISBN 978-3-033-08839-9

Contents

Introduction	7
Mountain Racer	13
In the Beginning	13
Zermatt	14
Early Racing	16
Experiencing the Inner Game	20
Learning to Feel	23
It's Child's Play	23
Theory Versus Feeling and Experiencing	27
Learning Through Experience	29
Connecting and Trust	32
Connecting	34
Mind over Matter	36
Feel It to Enjoy It	37
Overcoming Bad Habits with Feeling	38
Rhythm and Flow	40
Let Go to Get in the Flow	40
Being Free	42
Life on the Edge	43
Take it to the Limit	44
Stress	46

Staying in Control to Maintain an Edge	48
Flow in Day-to-Day Life	49
Awareness	53
Developing Awareness	53
Body Awareness	54
Becoming Aware	56
Present Moment Awareness	59
Meditation	61
Breakthrough	67
Autopilot	67
Second Wind	70
A Question of Balance	72
Overcoming Difficulties	75
What is a Breakthrough?	77
Being Reasonable	80
Both Sides of a Breakthrough	83
Flatland Breakthrough	85
The Mind	87
Focus	87
Break on Through	88
Visualization	92
What is Visualization?	92
If You Can See It, You Can Do It	94
Visualization—See it to Feel It	96
Inner Learning	98
Changing a Bad Mood to Good	99

Contents

Managing Fear	102
Nature of Fear	102
Beyond Fear	104
Moving on from Fear	107
Adrenaline Rush	110
Feeling Fear	114
The Moment Called Now	115
Being Present	115
Vision	118
How Being Present Creates a Personal Vision	119
Developing a Personal Vision	124
Character and Style	125
Personal Style	131
Principles of Presence and the Flatland	133
Breath in the Here and Now	135
One Breath In	136
The Journey is the Destination	138
The White Game	140
Acknowledgments	143

Introduction

The intensity of concentration required in competitive sports is a discipline beyond the physical demands of strength and balance. That single-pointed awareness can become a flow of continual attention that leads to a euphoric mental state known as a breakthrough. You can see it on the faces of the winning athletes on the podium as they reflect on this experience. The winner will smile and talk about being in a flow whereas the third-place finisher will shrug their shoulders and say they couldn't find a rhythm.

While breakthroughs are mostly associated with sports practitioners, this experience is not exclusively limited to athletic accomplishments. Also known as presence, this feeling of contentment and clarity can be experienced no matter what your background, discipline, or activity.

Being fully present in a natural state of fulfillment is one of the most satisfying and essential parts of our existence. We enjoy these moments when we are experiencing them but it's usually by chance rather than intent that we arrive there. The question then becomes: how do we learn to find our way to a place of contentment in the midst of our busy lives and what tools are available to let us effortlessly experience a more focused life?

Peter Kronig has been teaching his unique, practical techniques of living in the moment since the 1970s to guide people to a place of completeness and fulfillment. Even though Peter's profession is ski teacher, his approach is not limited to being on a mountaintop but something beneficial in everyday life.

The rush of speed and ecstatic high of winning are experiences Peter knows very well from his racing days as a ski champion. Exploring the principles behind his success, he was able to transfer his wisdom on how to be present to a variety of students over a long and successful career. These practical guidelines for living in a state of inner wellbeing unfold in this book as he shares stories and insights from the various stages of his life. Peter describes the path to presence as a process of moving from feeling the moment via all our senses to finding a rhythm and flow in our actions for an increased state of awareness and ultimately a breakthrough state of mind.

Introduction

Zermatt was the center for the winter jet set in the 1980s, and Peter was a much-in-demand instructor teaching celebrities ranging from rock stars to Academy Award-winning film directors. Tony Ashton, a musician who has played on sessions with George Harrison, Eric Clapton and Paul McCartney was an avid ski fan and performed every winter season in the legendary Hotel Post where Peter spent a lot of his evenings. In his autobiography, *Zermattitis,* he said Peter 'was regarded as the star of the Zermatt instructors and he reminded me of Rudolf Nureyev'. Later, in a more mature phase of teaching, Peter's clientele grew to include top leaders in the business universe, including bankers and CEOs with private teaching assignments that took him around the world to exotic ski locations.

Peter grew up in Zermatt but ventured out in his teens to spend the off-season working as a steward on cruise ships, traveling the world from Asia to South America and everywhere in-between. Later, in his twenties, he was a top model in Paris and New York, enjoying a glamorous life. While doing photo shoots and television ads he threw himself into the spirit of the Swinging Sixties, partying in exclusive clubs and dining with famous designers. He always came back to Zermatt every ski season and used his feeling-based approach to help students on their way to a breakthrough.

He had always skied, introduced to the sport at a young age by his father who was one of Switzerland's first certified teachers. He evolved into a successful local racer at his hometown of Zermatt and was invited to become a member of the Swiss national ski team. From watching top skiers race, Peter learned the principles of visualization, which allowed him to imitate the performance of the pros and win races.

I first met Peter when I moved to Switzerland and knew he was a ski teacher in Zermatt but not much more. We would cross paths at social events, and a couple of years ago he asked me to help write his story and share his knowledge. Over the course of many visits to his hometown in the shadow of the Matterhorn, we talked about some of his adventures and how his authentic teaching style had evolved. I was excited by the chance to help share the natural wisdom from his mountain life and down-to-earth know-how in developing awareness. Influenced by a lifetime of practicing meditation, his approach is all the more relevant given today's interest in the themes of mindfulness and conscious living.

Based on many conversations, the book is written in

INTRODUCTION

the first person to preserve Peter's natural expression in our meetings. It's like having a conversation with a good friend and trusted guide who shares their humor and simple insights. I hope you enjoy the wisdom and inspiration as much as I have. Peter has helped me to understand the preciousness of each moment, which made me realize that our conversations were not just about skiing and that there is no ultimate end goal, other than learning to live a full and rewarding life of continuous inner wellbeing.

Mountain Racer

In the Beginning

Learning to ski was like when I first started walking as a child. Usually, people can recall when they ski for the first time but I don't even remember. I was three years old. The furthest I can think back is when I broke my first skis. At that time, we only had wooden skis and the wood was dry and old so it just needed a little pressure to break. My father got me secondhand skis because they would never last very long. When I got to a point where I didn't like them I would ski into a bump and the tips would break away. Then I would get some other skis that were a little better. It was fun.

When I started out, I walked around in front of the house with my skis on, falling down and getting up laughing. But I didn't mind crashing—it was anyway just a game. I managed to practice on a little field in front of the house, falling down until I got the hang of it.

That's how learning happens. You do an exercise two or three times and then all of a sudden there is this one run where you don't fall. Amazingly enough, you pick it up very quickly. As a child, you become a specialist in learning. Even jumping with a little sled off a bump and turning over, you giggle. You don't judge yourself. Judging is for the grown-ups and falling really aggravates them. When it's a game you laugh about it.

That's why all the champions in sports or other disciplines have learned their skills when they were young. There's very little judgment and mental activity because it's a game. Awareness goes a long way because you can observe your awareness and speed up the learning as you see how your body and mind function. You might have an academic outlook but it originally started from being aware. It's the capability we have for whatever we're learning, whether it's physical or intellectual. If you're present and aware of awareness, then your learning capacity increases. You need to be open to it and not stick exclusively to a system or technique. You have to stay with what your senses are feeling to be present.

Zermatt

I wasn't really taught to ski, I just went with my father. He was in the first group that completed an exam to become a certified ski instructor in Switzerland in the mid-1920s. Around 1925 they started developing ice skating and skiing in Zermatt, and the Grand Hotel Zermatterhof made a small skating rink where my father would teach skating to the guests, and sometimes he also taught them skiing. During the war, there was no tourism and because he had a big family he started working as a conductor on the Gornergrat Railway.

I saw Zermatt change after the war from when we had mountain climbers in the summer to where it became a year-round resort. There were a lot of American soldiers visiting who were based in Germany. They would come for the week and go skiing in their uniforms and the local ski instructors taught them how to ski. We were little kids and would stop them on the street because we knew how to stretch out our hands and say "chewing gum." They would give us sticks of gum.

In the 1950s, there were a couple of races in Zermatt and some local heroes were on the Swiss national team. They participated in the regional FIS (International Ski Federation) races. These were the precursor to what became the official circuit—it was the early days before they had the rating system. The World Cup came later in the late 1960s.

The older skiers were a great example and while we were still in school we watched them training but mostly they were always going from race to race. I was one of two or three boys who dominated the school races and I usually wrecked three or four pairs of skis each season. That's from skiing every day for four-and-a-half to five months. We were completely hooked on skiing; it was the only thing we could do, that or sledding.

Early Racing

When I was twelve or thirteen I got my first really long racing skis from a racer in Zermatt. They were 215 centimeters long and I couldn't reach the tip when I stretched out my hand—it was that much taller than me. In the beginning, I had a hard time because they were dominating me more than I was controlling them. When I finally took control, there was a lot more stability and speed and I really started going. Nobody had ever taught me any techniques. I would watch the good skiers and imitate them.

I did well in the school races and when I was fifteen was chosen to race in the downhill at the championships of the Canton (county). These races originated in the Swiss army, with championships held every year in downhill, slalom, cross-country, jumping—everything. The race was in Crans-Montana and it was snowing like hell. At that time the goggles were not effective, so you couldn't see anything. I even crashed once during the race because of the conditions, and the run wasn't prepared, but I got up and continued. There were no gates, just little flags and I got to the finish. I was completely pissed off because it hadn't gone the way I wanted so I didn't even wait for the results. I went back to the little hotel where we were staying and an hour later somebody came and asked why I had left. I was totally surprised because even though I crashed once, I came in second.

At another championship of the Canton, I won the giant slalom and the slalom. I had gotten into such a flow, it was so incredible, and somehow I felt it even before I started. The man at the starting gate had to hold me as I couldn't wait to get going and I made the best time of the day. That was the strongest breakthrough I experienced when I was starting out. After that result, I was sent to the Swiss championships where I came in third in the slalom, and Roger Staub was first. (When they had the Olympics in Squaw Valley, he won a gold medal in the giant slalom.)

The first international races started with racers attend-

The White Game

ing from Austria, Italy, France, and Switzerland. In Zermatt, they had the Gornergrat Derby and all the top racers came—it was quite well-known. For this competition, I was in the slalom and I came in ninth among the ten best ones. That of course motivated me to get a little more into racing. When I was eighteen I won some local regional races in order to eventually join the Swiss national team. We didn't have helmets or safety bindings, no nothing, it was crazy. To fight against the wind resistance, we would put bands just below the knees so the pants wouldn't flutter. And we started wearing these thin, tight jackets which were very basic compared to what they wear today.

We went to a giant slalom in Austria where I was the first among the Swiss, reaching fifth place overall, which was a good international result. It's a great feeling. When you win a race, you know why. You know from the beginning that you're in a breakthrough and you keep the line, even exaggerating the speed, becoming more compact, and going for it. You feel it. As soon as I was through the finish and heard from the loudspeaker that it was the new record I wasn't even surprised because I felt that it was fast. It's probably the same in car racing or any kind of competition—you're 100 percent there.

Then you can win if you have the technique and the know-how.

The only trouble was that in the 1950s there was no money in racing. I would have continued but I gave it up because I couldn't afford it. I had to beg money from my father to pay for my trips. From when I was eighteen we started getting two pairs of skis from a well-known Swiss brand but beyond that, there was no support. You needed clothes and racks and all kinds of things. Today, the skiers make a lot of money and have big sponsors. The last time I raced I didn't have much training because I had already started working the previous summer as a steward on cruise ships going to the Caribbean or Montreal. The last race I did that winter was the championships of the Canton and I won the slalom again, but after that, I was more interested in traveling and seeing the world.

I started racing when I was fifteen and every year after the races were over, I got some clients from the ski school in Zermatt to make a little pocket money during the winter. In the beginning, I was helping out as an assistant instructor and didn't really know anything about teaching or technique. They never told me how I should teach or what to teach; in their heads, it was logical that I could teach since I was a good skier. My approach was very spontaneous and simple. The only thing I referred to was the contact of the skis with the snow, how to change the weight, and watching the inside and outside edges. With that, I was quite successful, but it was all completely unstructured. I didn't really know if it was going to go anywhere, but it actually worked. The people I skied with enjoyed it too because it was very simple, without a lot of theory, ideas or fear. As soon as they started feeling a little bit about what was going on, the length of their skis, and the edges, they became very confident. Because they were aware of what they were feeling, it pushed the fear away.

Experiencing the Inner Game

When I took the exam to be a certified ski instructor I learned everything by the book—the techniques and all the concepts around it. I passed my exam and did quite well but when I was skiing I didn't use any of that, I just used the feeling. On paper, we define what a parallel is, what a snow plow is. It's all broken up into intellectual subjects but it has nothing to do with what you're feeling because that's the real teacher. Technique is not awareness and experiencing.

Mountain Racer

Once I was certified and started teaching, I was using both approaches: awareness and theory. For almost ten years I sort of mixed the two, but it frustrated me because it wasn't as simple and pure as it was when I didn't focus on technique; one doesn't work with the other. That's why, at the beginning of my thirties, I thought about giving up teaching skiing.

Around that time, I went to the United States and at a conference heard Tim Gallwey speaking about the Inner Game (of Tennis). I was fascinated because it was a confirmation of why my teaching worked when I only used awareness. I was already close to the Inner Game principles with my experience-based approach. I introduced myself and later we talked about skiing and the Inner Game. That's the first time he considered doing a book on The Inner Game of Skiing but I couldn't participate because I was living in Switzerland. Later that year, I was invited to an Inner Game clinic for ski instructors in Boulder, Colorado.

When I got back to Switzerland I was inspired by what I had learned from some of the exercises but for me, it was still mostly about feeling. It was a good experience and it related to my breakthroughs in skiing. I believe in the system and it has helped me to be more conscious

The White Game

and look at my own experience a little deeper. And that's what restarted my joy of teaching, and I began to enjoy skiing again just as I did when I was racing.

After I returned I had a meeting with the official ski school committee in Zermatt where I introduced the Inner Game. They'd heard some background from one of the instructors I had talked to about it and said they wanted to meet with me. I could see after my presentation that they were not at all open to the concept, and one of the directors of the school said they had been doing it like that since the beginning. After the meeting they let me do my thing because I wasn't working in the school and had enough work without them with my own private clients. One of the committee members I knew wasn't there but was later briefed about the presentation, and he told them: "Peter is fifty years ahead of you."

I started to find out that when I left the theory out and only worked with the idea of "feeling" that the students relaxed and were having fun learning. It changes the whole atmosphere of what skiing is all about. It's like in day-to-day life when you're in that state of experiencing being present during what you do—then you can have fun.

Learning to Feel

It's Child's Play

The biggest advantage children have is that they are fearless. The greatest obstacle for grown-ups is being afraid. Even though adults say they have no fear, you can see when they have it because it's normal when standing on a steep mountain. They're more aware of the danger and the risk. In the back of their mind, they think: "What will happen if I am out for several weeks or even months because of an accident?" It makes them uptight. And when they fall down, they judge themselves or get mad and frustrated. When the experience of being present is there, you can be in control, take it easy and not ski over your head. That's an expression from ski technique. It means you don't ski with your head, your concepts, and go over your limit.

Skiing is a game for children because they're playing. For them, it is pure and natural. When you're in the playing

The White Game

mood, learning is automatically going on, whether consciously or not. Kids just go for enjoyment because that's what they're born with. It's amazing to see how quickly they copy you without needing much guidance. If you see they are scared, you just say "watch how I do it and see what it feels like." Then they do it without needing any explanations. When you explain something to kids it doesn't register, they don't really listen. All they want is to have fun. Natural fun. Since they're still present naturally, even if it's only 50 percent, they go for it and they let go. It becomes 100 percent a game.

Children love to ski without poles because then they need more balance. It's a challenge for them because it makes it more difficult. They love that. But when a grown-up is challenged, they get more scared instead of feeling safer. It's a game for the kids because they are in the presence and they play with it. When I was little we had very few lifts so the biggest game was taking a shovel and building a jumping hill out of snow. We would build it as high as we could and jump. The sensation is similar to walking to the top of a cliff and diving off. The kick is that second you spend in the air. I broke a number of skis jumping this way. Children love games like that.

Learning to Feel

Most instructors love to ski with kids because they don't have to make much of an effort, they're just playing with them and the children learn. You don't have to explain much to a child; they're not really interested. If you try, they just look around so you join in the game. The one thing they learn the most from is copying. It's very natural and automatic that kids imitate. Visualization, imitation, and copying are used by kids instinctively and they are the basic tools of awareness. In other words—they feel it.

Children have no fear because it's a game and when they fall, they laugh—it's fun and they're playing. That's why they're so high when they're very young. We all dream of the happiness that we experienced when we were children playing all the time. They are still in the here and now, and then we educate them and send them to school where they learn how to be absent. Instead of developing what we were born with, we developed our finite mind. The kids are always there in the flow but the older they get the more they start to think about everything. And the grown-ups have big problems with learning to ski because they only refer to the technique and don't feel anything. But when you get them to feel it right from the beginning, there are no obstacles—they

The White Game

get into it very quickly. The kids don't bother about technique; they are already learning from playful experience.

When I have a class of children, I try to get out of the way to let them find an experience on their own. I talk to them before starting to ski, and to make them aware of the danger I tell them things such as always watch the other skiers when they come close to you. You have to warn them of the hazards and to be careful because once children feel they have no fear they really let it go. It makes much more sense to the grown-ups when you talk to them about the risks. Children listen to you but they don't take much of it in because once they learn how to ski they love to go fast. After they've had a couple of good crashes without getting hurt, they become a little more sensible. They make their own experiences of almost crashing, of nearly running into somebody, and it teaches them. There is no wrong action, every mistake is teaching you.

When we're kids we're naturally in the world of feeling. We are present. It's important to be clear about what the feeling is and what understanding it and judging it is. With kids, there is no judging when they fall. They just laugh and get up and do it again and then they finally get it. It's very simple. It's natural. We're capable of feeling when we're born. We cry when we're hungry.

Theory Versus Feeling and Experiencing

I took the exam to become an instructor when I was twenty. We were given a book to learn the technical skills but my whole teaching approach came from feeling what you experience. I only referred to feelings when I taught and it worked, so I didn't think too much about it.

When I finally became an instructor using all the theory and the technique, I right away noticed that clients got confused. I thought that teaching by technique was the right thing to do and I tried to get used to it. I got frustrated having to explain what was right, what was wrong, what they should and shouldn't do. It was creating interference with the simple pure experience that comes through feeling.

But if I stopped teaching technique and stuck to awareness and the experience, everything happened and the clients were happy. They were getting high on it and learned very quickly. They had the sense they could change to what worked, not doing right or wrong, rather just focusing on a feeling. That's the a-ha experience kids normally have. We adults screw it up. I finally gave up trying to combine the two approaches when I taught. I just shared the experience of skiing. It always worked and still does.

Racers function by feeling and imitating the best skiers because that's the natural way we learn. It's not even a system, it's just witnessing what you experience and expressing what you observe. That then creates feedback in the memory banks. Once we feel we can do it, there's a breakthrough, it becomes real. It's very easy because you don't need any theory.

As soon as you do exercises like feeling the snow, the student starts to develop their awareness. People are blown away because it's not only that they can ski, they feel it works. And in finding the presence is that joy. The more you feel it, the deeper you go.

Teaching through awareness and feeling eliminates the technical part because the technicalities can become an obstacle. Learning through awareness has no negative aspect. It's totally natural. Using that approach would simplify the ski school teaching tremendously. It would be much more effective and people would have more fun. Some people get so frustrated that they don't continue skiing. They get frustrated because they take it apart and intellectualize, which becomes an obstacle. When you're in your head, there is no learning taking place and it becomes a form of aggravation.

Learning Through Experience

In a ski school, the instructors have to follow a structure so they can certify students at a level to do the specific techniques. The methodology is important as it is a system of control. We must have control but it's not the ultimate approach, it's not the secret. The only thing that teaches the secret is experience. And if you really get into the depths of the experience then you come to the point where you don't need the technique anymore because the experience holds everything. The more you do it, the better you get.

Technique is structured to give students knowledge. But then they need to experience skiing with an instructor who gives them the possibility to ski with awareness. Then there's gratitude when a student finishes a difficult run and that gives them a certain self-respect. The gratitude that they can ski such a course and do something they have never dreamed of. The feeling that everything is possible simply by being in the present moment.

You don't reach a limit when going deep into what you

experience; you can always go further. Because you have been conscious of life you can appreciate what being in the moment really holds. It's a very interesting thing because it can really go in every direction whether you ski or not—you'll never come to the finish line. The joy and the fulfillment will also grow.

Jean-Claude Killy, the first World Cup alpine ski racer, said in an interview after a big World Cup win: "As long as I can feel the contact with the snow I can do anything and when I lose that feeling of the presence I risk crashing." All top skiers, when they get to a finish with a good result, refer to the feeling, not the technique.

When you tell a class to feel the snow and apply it, and then ask the students afterward what they felt, they would all have different observations. Like the snow was pretty hard, here it was soft, very good snow, slippery. It doesn't really matter what they experienced but it's proof to me that they did feel the snow. What they felt is not really important because if they feel it, that means they're present. Learning is happening. They are in contact with the element—that's the important thing.

Some people would react very euphorically and say this is great, skiing like this works. Another would say they didn't really feel any difference from before. It all

Learning to Feel

depends on how they explain what they're feeling, the mood they are in, and whether it felt good. Maybe it was just very subtle so they didn't get too excited. At the beginning, others would also say "I can't feel anything." Then I tell them to keep trying because you must be feeling something even standing still. They would say "yeah, I feel my skis" or "my feet" or something. I would ask if they could feel something underneath? "Yeah, I can feel the snow." All of a sudden, they realize that they can actually feel the snow. Then it has to be practiced. You practice that and automatically start getting more secure because you are in contact with the snow which is the most important thing. Once they know the quality of connecting to the snow then they automatically stick to it. And probably they'll continue to ski that way for the rest of their life. Once you get into it and have a certain depth of experience, that's the proof that it works. I can feel the snow, I can feel the angulation of the edges and notice how I control it, and the overall experience becomes much more functional.

You always go back to something that works—it's the negative stuff you try to get rid of. Bad habits are usually things people do because they are not conscious. They are not feeling anything. Then it blows up into a concept and they don't even know what they are doing wrong. When they have experienced the snow and the quality of it, then they let go of what doesn't work because you always go for what works. It's the same in whatever you do.

Connecting and Trust

As a teacher, I try to connect with the student by focusing them on feeling the sensations their body provides. If a student manages to get into the feeling of their actions, it produces know-how. They can feel that's how it works even though they know they have to practice to control it. They experience that it functions, and trust automatically comes in as well as joy because they can feel it working. They are open to learning because they have a result—it's not theory, it's an experience. It simplifies teaching.

They build up their desire to practice and go skiing and want to learn how to increase that feeling. Even if that experience is very little, it's strong enough that it'll make them hungry and they'll want more and more. At the same time, it makes them thankful because the teacher showed them how. They also see that as a teacher I can only guide them but they have to do it themselves. It's

Learning to Feel

the same as wanting to change this world—we all have to do it as an individual. That's the relation of student and teacher.

I can look at a person and see that he doesn't really know whether he's enjoying it or not. They're thinking this run looks very difficult, and maybe they're not ready to take the time and will only experience frustration trying to learn this. To overcome that, you have to help them concentrate on what they're doing. They begin to sense that it's a game and start to feel that edge where the ski makes contact with the snow. They also get a lot of energy from it because the energy comes in immediately from being present. When you start to experience by letting go and just feeling that edge, you use very little energy.

The beginner students feel it when it starts to function and they have that a-ha experience. They know if they practice it, they could do it like these other skiers around them and that's what they want. It establishes trust to be able to control their skiing. It's there in whatever we do—whether it's sports or day-to-day life. It's always the same thing, just in different fields. The emotions, the liking, and the joy are always here in the heart. Contentment.

The White Game

Connecting

My teaching approach is that experience is the teacher. And the mind is the mind; it's the judgment. The joy is in the experience. You might need the mind because you want to know the results you get in a race but it doesn't have anything to do with the experience.

Skiing is a very unnatural thing at the beginning when you start, especially as a grown-up, because you haven't practiced it before. You slide when your weight is in the wrong place and you fall and that can be aggravating. You have to tell people right at the start of the class that they will fall but not to worry. If you don't go too fast and you're relaxed, you'll be OK. Falling is part of the process and when you tumble, you haven't done anything wrong. It's just another experience that will teach you.

Once you start falling, the skis react in a very natural way, but if you fight it, you become stiff. If you let go you might avoid the crash and at least you are relaxed, so it diminishes the possibility of getting hurt. When students have had that experience and later get into other situations, they start feeling: "I have to be careful now because otherwise, I'm going to go into the area where I can fall." It's all about learning through feeling.

Learning to Feel

By doing it right comes the joy and then you want to do it better. You learn not to take so much risk the next time and then you can get through that stretch of the mountainside without crashing.

I've seen a lot of people get annoyed because the instructor said: "don't do that, that's wrong," judging them. That's an incorrect attitude because every mistake is also teaching you. But if you stick to awareness, you'll enjoy it. You'll fall and you'll be sitting in the snow and you're laughing. You're not hitting the snow with your sticks because you're mad that you couldn't do it. Awareness is a big thing but the source of it is small and simple. Enjoyment is important in our life.

Learning to feel your actions is not that complicated and you'll benefit because if your awareness grows, you can use it in whatever you do in life. And at the same time, we become intoxicated by joy so it develops the depth of our happiness. Instead of being aggravated like an angry politician, you can play and move through the mountains and be happy. You don't have to take it seriously, it's just a game, a beautiful game and that's it. That's why people get very hooked on skiing. You're out in the open and the air is good and you're on vacation, you're relaxed. And if you can go deeper into the relaxation, it can become, as the French say: *Magnifique*. Watch how much fun kids have playing their games; they don't care whether they fall or not because they're 100 percent into what they're doing. Life for them is still a game, they haven't gotten to the point where we make everything so serious. It's not really so serious.

Mind over Matter

When you feel the snow, the pressure, and the speed, automatically your thinking process is in motion too. We always talk to ourselves and even comment on our actions. When something feels good we tell ourselves in our head: "Oh, this is nice, I have to keep doing that to enjoy it." That's where we use the mind but the trouble is when it dominates us then disaster is very close. With our mind or intellect, we are conscious of what we're doing and it can be analyzed. If we want to learn, it comes automatically by referring to the experience of what we're doing because that's what's teaching us. You can program the mind by saying that was good. Experience and thinking are hooked up. It's automatic, we've had it for a long time.

The mind is there to acknowledge the experience and judge it. It's good, it's bad, but the teacher is the feeling.

Learning to Feel

We have both. The more we become aware, the more we relax, the more the natural teacher takes over the teaching part. The mind becomes the observer but it also judges, which can drive you crazy. When we're in a state of stress, we're totally in our minds. When you're 100 percent in your mind, you can't feel anything anymore and then you experience pressure and stress.

The mind has its purpose. We have to think, we have to decide, but that should be a tool of feeling. Humanity isn't there yet but I think evolution is going that way. It's experience that has taught us what functions and what doesn't. We have gone so far with technique and science that the mind takes on the role of acknowledging what we can feel. It shouldn't be there to judge if something is wrong or right. In sports, you have to first refer to the feeling.

Feel It to Enjoy It

Sylvain Saudan was the first person to ski down the face of many of the world's tallest mountains like Mont Blanc and Mount McKinley as well as a lot of high peaks in the Himalayas. He's considered the father of extreme skiing for his many pioneering steep descents. The French call him "The Skier of the Impossible." He once said:

The White Game

"I can't think when I ski. The only thing I do is feel and enjoy." When you feel with the edges of your skis and the sensation of the contact with the snow, there's feedback to your memory banks and learning takes place. When you only think, there is zero feedback and you experience confusion, instability, and fear. Heightened awareness only happens when you know how to let go of your mind. Which means feeling. When you're present the energy flows—you don't only use energy, you're also recharged. When you start thinking, you block the recharging system. What follows is that you feel out of balance—you feel fear and panic. When people start thinking, they lean back and get afraid and nothing is happening because they cannot control the skis. After all, they're too far back. You're blocked, there's nothing you can do.

Overcoming Bad Habits with Feeling

To overcome limitations from bad habits you need to consciously look at the pattern. Become conscious of what it feels like and then go to the feeling. You have to work with students so they really experience what's going on with their bad habits. Feeling it correctly is a different experience than when you do something

Learning to Feel

wrong. The habit limits their progress—they just do it because it's a routine. You tell them what to concentrate on, what to feel, and then they have a comparison. They see it works much better, feels much better, and then they give up the old practice. Once they experience something new that makes it easier, then they go for it. The bad habit is gone. You have to create a feeling for what works.

Once you experience something that works, then you let go. That's how you progress. It's all through feeling. You might fall back but you know what to concentrate on so it functions. If all of a sudden you get stiff or tired, and you're in your head instead of the feeling, then things start to go wrong, even with a good skier. Then you just let go and feel your edge, the angle of your ski and go for it. Then feeling happens again and you get back into the rhythm.

It's again the same thing—be conscious, relax, feel what you do. Don't be absent by thinking about your problems or how you're skiing. You should be concentrating on the skiing. Be here now. It's always the same. Awareness. Feeling. When you feel, you're present; when you think, you're absent.

Rhythm and Flow

Let Go to Get in the Flow

Feeling your actions leads to finding a rhythm and flow that becomes a breakthrough. The rhythm has two phases. First, you feel it starting to happen and you sense right away that things are going better. Then when you let go of that, you go even deeper into a flow and that's when everything comes together and the racer wins. To experience the flow, you have to let go completely. When you're in that rhythm it makes you very high because it's the presence. Once you're in that rhythm, the more you experience it, the more you trust it, the more you will relax into it. Sometimes it's almost an out-of-body experience. You feel that you're skiing well and you're right there in the present moment. That's when you have a very good result, that's the breakthrough.

When you feel the breakthrough, that feeling of being in a flow, you totally let go to it because you know you

Rhythm and Flow

can play with it. That's when you go one step further. You don't concentrate on your technique or anything like that, you just groove on the flow. When you're in that rhythm, in that total presence, the more you do it, the better you get.

In a slalom race, you first study the course. It's short and has many quick turns so you have to be very concentrated. Then, when you're at the starting gate, you let go completely so when you race, the rhythm is there. It takes you right to the presence. And when there is the slightest thought during the slalom course, you're already out. If you stay right there in the flow, then it gets very strong. Sometimes your mind comes up and says "watch it" and that's enough to fall. When you let go, you don't have to remember difficult gates where you have to be careful. Once you're in the flow nothing is happening, you're amazed at what you're feeling. It's total presence. The result is constantly there, it's the breakthrough.

After a race, they always interview the first two or three skiers. You watch the one who won and before he starts talking you can see he's completely elated. The guy who's second or third: "I had difficulty on the first ten gates because I couldn't get into the rhythm." That's enough to lose half a second. What's interesting is you can feel right away when you're in the flow. When you train for slalom, for example, after two or three years of racing you know the flow. You know exactly what to do at the start and that's to feel the contact with the snow.

Being Free

We're told we have to work a certain way, or work for a company and behave according to their standards—that's the way society is structured. Along with the expectations of our parents, these could all be technical limitations on a personal level. It's important to balance these expectations with finding your way forward in order to be free from the technical confines.

You're only free when you're on that edge. When you ski or listen to music then you're present, then you start flowing. It always comes back to the center—be here now. When you become a little conscious from practicing meditation and start to develop it more, that's the place where we have to learn to be and to practice it to be in sync, otherwise, we are just derailing.

When you practice being present and look out from that viewpoint, then the technical is absolutely OK. What we have done with science and technology is sensational.

Rhythm and Flow

You can use it to function so that everything works. Today it looks like we're lost in the technology and fascinated or absorbed by it. But it controls us instead of us controlling it. We have to come to the point in evolution where we can really understand and use technology. To be able to look at it and use it to its full potential we need to be in that place of presence, the here and now.

Life on the Edge

To start the journey of finding a flow, you begin by feeling the snow, and for that the edges of the skis are tools. From there you have to adapt your performance to what you're feeling. It's accepting what's there, letting go, and with your knowledge about skiing, playing with it. That's how you get into it. The feedback comes from feeling the edges. Then when you're in a flow and ski on a familiar run, you're present. You become very aware of the surroundings like the landscape; you're not just strictly skiing. Awareness is much bigger. Even though you're present when you go down a hill, at the same time you can watch the view and see down below that there's a forest. It's as if it comes second to what's happening, but you actually experience a lot more when you're in the feeling and find a flow. I've noticed that, especially when I ski on my own. On the difficult part of a ski run my concentration is really focused on what is right there. But as soon as it gets easier, I become aware of all the surroundings: the temperature, the snow condition, and even what I'm hearing where the tone becomes harmonious. It all becomes very beautiful and reaches a breakthrough level. Joyful. Since the presence is open to everything that increases the joy and adds to that natural high.

Skiing is a constant adapting to the snow. There are no two turns that follow that are alike. Even when you ski slalom, which consists of very short turns, even though they look exactly the same, they are different. Each turn is a unique feeling. And when you start to notice these details you automatically train your awareness to be present. The reward is very good—it's joy. Fulfilling. It's not a joy you want to show off. It's that feeling you cannot really communicate—it's beyond words. You become one with the experience—that's another dimension of the breakthrough of perfection.

Take it to the Limit

Taking it to the limit is when you are on the edge of the ski. When you're at an angle of 90 degrees that's the

Rhythm and Flow

thinnest amount of contact with the snow and you're still managing to stay in control and achieve the highest speed. Being on the edge at 90 degrees is where the breakthrough is possible, that's where it happens. We're on that edge, that element of perfect control, when we walk and move around. Whatever we do, our body has to function and it does it very well. By practicing being present, we'll start to have the understanding that when we are awake we are on that edge all the time. Probably even when we're asleep because we are breathing.

There is the visual world and there's the creative world, our life. That's where we have to start. That's why we talk so much about being present, being in the flow. It probably takes many years to be able to understand where we come from, how we function, and who our true self is. It's also why we feel so excited and high when we get into the presence, listening to some beautiful music, and start flying. Being in the moment needs to be practiced to have that understanding. It has to be a conscious act all the time so we can grow. That's why it's quite difficult to talk about things that profound because it goes beyond words. You can look at it from the perspective of understanding, and that's how you become conscious.

Stress

When you're losing your edge, you're hanging one way or the other. That's also how our mood goes. When we get stressed and then have a conscious breath we can look again at the situation and not get enslaved by the stress. That's when we become conscious of how we can overcome stress and learn to look at ourselves whatever happens in life, whether we ski or work in an office. When we get into something rhythmic like music, we let go automatically because it pleases us and we start flying with it. There's a lot of joy and the proof is there that it doesn't take a lot of effort to feel it. It's very important to remember that we always go up and down. If your consciousness grows and you become aware of that, then we really start handling stress. There is so much theory and anxiety about how to manage it. If stress comes we want to use a theory to manage it and it's not going to work. You have to be present to be able to look at yourself. The key is to take that deep breath and look at what's going on instead of being drowned in worry. We can look at it and build a picture of it and it looks very complicated but the process of becoming conscious is extremely simple. We have to know what this breath is all about and then it will happen.

Rhythm and Flow

Breath neutralizes you like a reset and then you're able to be present. When you're conscious of your breath the anger and frustration go away. It's the law of physics—two things cannot occupy the same place at the same time. The breath makes you conscious as it's the only thing happening at that moment because if you stop breathing that's the end of the game. Remember that breath and you're back in the moment. If you're in the now then you're not frustrated about what happened or angry about what could happen, you're just dealing with what is. It neutralizes the situation instead of your getting emotional about it. That isn't to say you can't have emotions but rather learning to manage the quality of the emotion. Not being dragged around by them which is where the mind comes in. Then it all starts snowballing, starts rolling, and then to wind it back up is more difficult.

Our emotions start working when things get difficult and then you're dominated by the emotional noise. To be able to look at it we have to learn how to let go. Go back to the presence and it's put aside. We should check that our emotions don't possess us—it's actually very simple. That's what we practice when we meditate. If the day comes where we can be cool and really look at ourselves, then our lives can be more pleasant. It can be really sensational. If the average human could raise their consciousness, this would help create a wonderful world.

We are always on the edge living in the moment called "now." Once we leave the mountaintop, we can have problems, but if we are on that edge then we are OK. It's a very fine line and we can feel it. Everybody's feeling it but not everybody's conscious of it. And to develop that awareness, that's the big secret. It always goes back to knowledge of yourself; it's always that edge. Stay there. We have trained ourselves to think we are controlling everything, but we're not—that's why we have so many problems.

Staying in Control to Maintain an Edge

To stay in control and in the flow is similar to riding a bicycle. It's that balance that takes over as soon as you're rolling. You're moving along and it's a very pleasant feeling. It's that edge, the balance, and everything is in sync. When we're driving a car it's not as joyous as on a bicycle but as long as we're in motion it feels great. Sitting in a car and rolling along, we can think about things. You can be driving a car and be happy because it's really great scenery, or you can be totally destroyed by your mind and be in a bad mood with problems and worries. All that can be neutralized the more you live on the edge or in the here and now—all these names, descriptions. The secret is to feel your actions without thinking. Since I've been working on this book project, feeling has become more important for me than my whole career of skiing. I'm getting into it when I'm talking about it and reaching a certain depth of feeling—it's the best. That's how you get to experience joy. We talk about a lot of other things but it's always the same. Like drinking something good or eating something we like. It shows us that we're in that presence when we feel what we taste, the satisfaction we get out of it, the energy we receive from it. It's the edge.

Flow in Day-to-Day Life

If I'm going to work, present in the act of doing my job, then my brain shuts down and I'm in the flow. Being in the flow is neutralizing any chatter because to maintain the flow you have to keep the momentum of the effort.

There are days you come into the office to do your work and everything just flows, everything works. Other days, nothing works because you're not there in the present moment or you're only partially there while also losing yourself in thoughts about the past or future. It depends on your state of mind—mind over matter. Every top skier experiences these moments and you don't even know why it's happening. You went to bed early, you slept a lot, you're eating healthily and you go out on the mountain and nothing works well. It functions but you don't get in a rhythm. It's because of some kind of absence. Probably your head is more with your girlfriend than your skis—it needs so little space. The mind only needs a little opportunity and it just takes over and buries you in a disaster. Then other times you haven't even slept much, you feel tired but then you had a good breakfast. You go out there and have no expectation whatsoever. You're going out training and running some gates and all of a sudden you feel that everything works even though you didn't sleep much. It depends on what mental state you're in.

When you're in the office engaging your senses in the world around you, it's like the feeling of the snow when you ski. It grounds you into that moment. You're connecting with the elements in an office environment; you've engaged your senses. In your day-to-day life you're not challenging why something is a certain way,

Rhythm and Flow

it's just what it is and you're only observing it.

All you're noticing when you are in a mental state is that you don't really feel like working because of some reason. You probably don't even know what it is, you're just in a bad mood. It's the same when you feel the snow. If you're in a bad mood you probably don't get into a rhythm very quickly. It bothers you and you don't even know what's bothering you. The sun is shining, the snow is perfect, life is good but you're in a bad mood and you're not happy—why? You of course have the choice when you know what to do. Do some breathing, do some yoga and it will bring you back to the presence. Relax a little bit and you feel a little joy and then it's fine again.

Even with unpleasant work that has to be done, with the right focus it doesn't bother you anymore. It always comes back to learning to let go. All you do is listen or feel—it's subtle. The more you practice presence, the better you get at it. It's like practicing skiing, the more you practice, the better you get. If you're relaxed and you do the work that needs to be done, you don't let it affect you because you're living in the moment—it's like a rhythm. It becomes flowing and you do it and once it's done it feels good; I can do that. It's self-control. On the

The White Game

other hand, what do we control? The key is the letting go. I like the expression in French, *lâcher prise*, which means to let go.

Once I was reading the Alcoholics Anonymous recovery program—a friend of mine was an alcoholic who attended AA. I was reading two or three pages of their program and they say, before doing anything, it's important to let go of everything, be neutral. They also use the power of breathing. Just breathe in a very relaxed way and let go. When you do this and you feel something pleasant then you automatically start feeling a little bit, even if it's just a small amount, of joy. You feel relaxed because you're not aggravated the way you are when you're looking for a solution to a problem. If you just do a little bit of breathing to let go, as soon as you experience the breath, you are recharged. The energy comes in and you're peaceful, your mood changes. It's a great tool, that breath. It's the secret to everything. and there probably is a lot more to unfold—we have only so far just scratched the surface. It's a miracle because it's what gives us life. Happiness comes out of the letting go. When we empty our mind then it can manifest itself. When we are in our head there is no room for it.

Awareness

Developing Awareness

It's very simple: feeling creates awareness. When you feel, you're present and it creates awareness in whatever you're doing, whether you're playing a musical instrument or skiing. Whatever you're working on you can get into a rhythm from being in the moment. When it's thinking work like mathematics or writing, it's difficult at the beginning, but then you get into a rhythmic flow. When there is rhythm there is feeling, and that creates awareness. Awareness is just a name. It comes when you are good at something, whatever it may be, whether you are performing on stage or doing sports. Even with writing, you get into it by watching your handwriting, and that's presence. That creates awareness. You're aware of breaking through. You're aware when you start dominating your subject and get into the flow. It's very simple. We have it as children when we play a game.

The more you do it, the better you get. You will have a breakthrough the more you're present and fully integrated with your actions.

I would tell students to get into what they're feeling by asking if they were aware of the temperature or the mountains around us. I got them into the feeling of their boots, their arms, their breathing and then we would focus on feeling the edges of their skis. The result was: "I'm feeling the snow and somehow I have gotten into the awareness thing and it works." All that is part of developing feeling.

Body Awareness

Body awareness is a very good practice for skiing or cultivating awareness in general. It's good to consciously move your body a little bit before you start skiing. Your elbows, your knees, your hips, to make sure you're there and not still at breakfast. When you want to go out skiing but the other part of you is thinking about your business, you do body exercises while feeling, so you're present. It also warms you up because it's cold and you shouldn't get off the lift half frozen and then immediately go full blast. Your body might not be ready to do that as your reaction time is not 100 percent; it's only

Awareness

80 percent and that can be fatal. It's part of a conscious warming up.

Being aware of your physique is something you learn that you have to do when you start skiing. Your physical condition will trigger questions in your head such as "am I ready to do this?" To ski or not to ski at that point. Some people jump off the plane after arriving from another continent and head up a mountain. They go from 1500 meters altitude up to 3000, thinking they can react just like they do at sea level, and that's not so. You have to be aware and know your body has to be loosened up, warmed up, in condition before you start doing anything.

When you start with a beginner you teach them to experience walking and the sliding it creates. They're not used to awareness movements so they're uptight and tense, and they get tired very quickly. But then by doing the movements they loosen up. That's also part of awareness. Awareness is the key for getting ready to go do something that demands a little more body-consciousness. It's again back to the what, the experience, what the feeling is. It's so complete that when you engage in your real life while you're in the presence it's very healthy.

The White Game

Most people can feel it when they just do light sports to be in condition and to be happy. "It's very important that I do these exercises that help me to concentrate when I'm working." It's good for your head, your body and even for your soul. We're made to move whether we walk or ski—it doesn't really matter which one.

When beginners start skiing, they're automatically stiff. When you start, it's almost like walking but because you're on skis you start sliding. You're doing something that is not natural like walking. You become curious about the movement because the experience has already started. I'm in motion but not by walking, by sliding, which happens automatically. The more you slide with nothing to stop you, the more likely you'll fall a couple times, but you won't get hurt. Then when you learn how to make a change of direction, it makes you high because you control it. We talk about having a breakthrough as an end result but the breakthrough actually starts much earlier with small victories.

Becoming Aware

Developing awareness starts with getting into the feeling of what your senses are telling you, and by focusing on that your mindfulness grows. Your experience becomes

Awareness

the focus because you're aware of the sensations of the environment. And we're also able to apply that to other scenarios. The input from whatever the stimulus is helps us begin to identify the feelings, and by making that a conscious action it then becomes awareness. It's one of the steps of getting into a flow. It's one name but you can also call it consciousness because that's also being aware.

Consciousness is the step after awareness when you make a conscious decision to do an action. It is, for lack of a better word, thoughtful. You're aware of things and able to make a mindful decision based on your awareness. You're making your choice from all the input you get. It's like in skiing when you're flying down the hill and decide to go right instead of left around a mogul because you can see the line down the mountain better. That's a conscious decision but it all happens so quickly, it's almost intuitive. The body has the intelligence to act, especially the balance.

When you make a conscious decision, your whole body aligns to fulfill that choice. It comes from awareness of this kind: "I am aware that it looks kind of rocky and over there is actually snow." You're aware of the snowfield and you make the conscious decision to steer clear

The White Game

of the rocks. Or maybe you think "I'm a macho, I can ski between the rocks." The choice to take the less dangerous route is actually not the mind because the mind might get in the way and then you start having a debate and by then it's too late.

You practice awareness by feeling. The more you concentrate on the sensations your body is experiencing, the clearer it gets because it's real. In skiing, it's when you start to feel the snow and you know the feeling of the downhill ski and the uphill ski or the outside edges and the inside edges. It's all about the contact with the element, the snow, and then you're present. When you're present, learning takes place and you also feel that it functions. It's like another a-ha experience which is very subtle, very simple. You start to remember how you started skiing as a kid when you were not even interested in what you were feeling. The only thing that counted was having fun, playing the game.

Awareness would simplify any kind of learning. You need your head to do mathematics and once you know the system it can be fun. It's like these youngsters beating the big champions at chess because they don't think about it. They make spontaneous moves and the guy opposite who has been playing thirty years calculates.

And the expert freaks out because they don't know why the opponent made a move. To become clear and understand what the experience teaches us is a great game. It's not a big philosophical, mathematical or some kind of a mind trip, it's real.

When we learn from experience it's magical because you open the door to rhythm and breakthrough. That's why the racers always talk about "I didn't get into the rhythm" or "I had a complete breakthrough." It's only through feeling that you get to that rhythm, which becomes a breakthrough, which is ecstatic. It really completely fulfills you because you are in total harmony with what you're doing and the elements. It's not hard being in harmony, it's just exciting.

Present Moment Awareness

Presence is a very important aspect right from the beginning through to even skiing in challenging conditions like deep snow. There you have to use your body weight but not be uptight because if you're uptight the edges will catch and you will fall more easily. When you're totally relaxed and your angle over the skis is right, then it becomes very harmonious and effortless. Then you get a lot less tired. That's when you can call it a dance.

The White Game

When you always go to the limit of your ability then it's very possible at a certain stage you will start to use a little strength instead of flowing. It just tightens you up and the danger of catching an edge is much bigger. That's why you should never go over 80 percent of your ability. When you use only a little energy, you enjoy it more. Body tension comes in very easily the closer you get to the maximum risk. It comes in quietly, you don't hear it, you don't notice it because you're in motion.

Some people give the feeling of harmony the name "embracing the mountain." I'd rather put it: enjoy the mountain. It's part of the awareness of the surrounding nature. When you feel all the details then automatically the mountain is included. Your whole environment is limitless. It's actually quite amazing what you can do through awareness. When you're in a total flow and at the same time aware of all the beauty of the mountains, the sun, and the motion, you're right in it. You're aware of it because you're present. You don't only feel, you also see it.

Awareness and being present are different words that have practically the same meaning. The more you let go, the more you are in the presence. It makes your consciousness grow and the more you let go it opens up the experience of presence—up to 100 percent. Then you're definitely in a rhythm or a flow and even a breakthrough. It makes you more conscious because you find something which is deep in that experience. It's very simple—there's no need to get into the different expressions of what consciousness or awareness or being present is. Our mind is very capable of turning letting go into a concept. We have to watch it because feeling and thinking about something is different. Whether it's consciousness or being present, feeling, letting go—it's all in one thing. It's complete. The more you practice it, the more it grows, the deeper you go, and the better it becomes.

Meditation

We have this habit of making meditation very philosophical and a lot of people like that. They're into beautiful names. But those names don't communicate the true value of the source where inner peace comes from. It's just names, going from one name to the other, and then we don't know anymore which comes first, consciousness or experience. It's actually much easier, it's just something that's happening in the presence and for that there's nothing like the breath. Then it happens.

The White Game

Why and how—it's not really interesting. We shouldn't analyze it, we should just enjoy it. Letting go is the biggest secret. The more you can let go when you practice meditation, the more beautiful it gets. It's not that easy but it has to be practiced. Like anything else, the more you practice, the more it becomes clear that something so simple, so beautiful can resolve everything. That's why it's so beyond words. The feeling has no words.

When I look at my life since 1975, which was when I first started to meditate, I have completely changed. When I look at my contentment, my fulfillment, my being at peace inside, I have completely transformed in a positive way. Peacefulness, contentment, being free—there are a lot of names but they are only names. Meditation is really an experience that has no system, no philosophy. It's just the breakthrough from focusing on your breath that will open into the divine dimension—no mantra, no nothing, just breathing. It has to be practiced to enter that place. There has to be a conscious desire to want to know, even if you don't know what it is. With conscious breathing, we are searching deep within, for that freedom, that liberty. The biggest secret of all secrets is in the breath. And once you are open to what it can bring, you practice it. When you go

Awareness

deeper in your practice, the joy becomes divine. Like the Chinese master Lau Tzu said: "Knowing others is intelligence; knowing yourself is true wisdom." That's it. It's simple, it's clear.

You can't really plan "I'm going to have a breakthrough this afternoon. I'm going to ride my bike in the beautiful countryside and find a flow." It will or it won't happen. It's like meditation. When you manage to let go completely you feel part of the oneness of all creation. And that's a breakthrough too. That's the divine breakthrough, to become one with the feeling of your own life energy. But how are you going to describe it if you don't experience it yourself? You can practice presence and eventually you will break through and then that understanding happens.

When we are having a good meditation, we can also start thinking about certain things we have to do, and all of a sudden there comes a moment of frustration. You just have to take a deep breath and focus again and it's OK. It's letting go. When we practice meditation, all we do is conscious breathing or when we do conscious skiing, it's also a feeling. When you feel, you're present; when you think, you're gone. There is no dogma, no theory—it's all about feeling, that's all. Meditation is like a breakthrough because it's also feeling. What is what doesn't really matter in the end. We have life, so we can groove on that and that's what we're learning. It's amazing.

A breakthrough is a part of what some people call samadhi. It's just a name, a different name. If you define samadhi as being at a high level of contentment and oneness with the world, it's very similar. A student once asked his master, "What is samadhi," and he answered, "It's like going to sleep without sleeping." That's meditation. It's beautiful. What it really means is this universe is infinite. We discover that there is a part of us that's infinite but we don't have the faintest idea where it starts. But it's fascinating. By using awareness, feeling, and working with our fear, we come to a breakthrough.

People feel it when you are relaxed and in the feeling of the presence in whatever you're doing. It's really beyond words because the feeling is so much stronger than any words—you can feel it, but you can't explain it. By practicing meditation, that understanding comes practically from being in the moment. It's an evolution. We practice it because we enjoy it and when we go inside there's probably no end to it. That's where the joy, the harmony, and the contentment lie, that's where the

Awareness

caring is—everything.

When you do it every day you become more conscious, more aware. It's something individual, just feeling. Presence is again one of those words when we feel something. It's an automatic process of how we function. When we feel, we're present. And when we think, we're in our mind and everything goes wrong. We get aggravated and end up in a bad mood.

There was a long period when I was young where skiing was an unconscious experience, but then, through focusing on awareness and especially meditation, I became clearer and more aware of my actions. It's where you're completely open and you can feel exactly what is teaching you—presence—feeling the element. Seeing it, hearing it, feeling, even tasting it when you eat snow.

I was already teaching people awareness when I started practicing meditation and understood the place of that in my approach. It made me very clear what had been happening without being conscious of it. I was feeling the snow without really knowing that was doing the trick.

When I was practicing presence, the more I did it the more I also started to realize it in other parts of my life. Experience is hooked up into this rhythmic feeling.

The White Game

There comes a point when you talk about presence where you have to stop talking because it's not about the words. It goes beyond words. When you practice presence, it becomes so fulfilling. You always enjoy it but joy takes on another dimension of understanding, fulfillment, and clarity. You see very clearly that's the way it is. It gives you a lot more acceptance. You get so clear that you feel joy. That's what we're all designed to be hooked up to, this enjoyment. It's natural. We want to be in this place and the more you practice presence the more you will enjoy life. And when you keep doing it, there is an evolution. It becomes more and more real because we see we are existing with our head controlling us instead of us controlling our head. It's about unlearning from being complicated and learning to be practical, simple, and real.

There are times when you're frustrated with yourself because you screw up things by using your head. And then it becomes clear—just stick to what you've always felt. It also changes you so that you become more aware and accepting. There's nothing to be frustrated about; anyway, it's a game. And it's real. It's the real game.

Breakthrough

Autopilot

Autopilot is just another name to describe finding presence. The best autopilot is breathing and because it's automatic we don't have to push a button. When you become conscious of your breathing, you're feeling what's going on in the present moment, knowing how to perfectly perform an action. Autopilot is the mechanism where you're in the flow and reach a state where everything is functioning without your having to think about it. That place of being where your body is in a state of mind where you don't need to make decisions because everything happens automatically.

Autopilot in skiing is when you feel the snow, you're present and the body works on its own by keeping the balance because there's constant change—every turn and every meter is different. The surface of the snow is not like a highway, it's not paved, it's constantly changing. And when you feel the snow, the rest of the body finds its equilibrium, like riding a bicycle. It's automatic, you don't have to think about it.

There's a part of autopilot in our balance that is natural in the way it functions. It's really quite amazing because if you take a couple of steps on a stairway while carrying something, the balancing of the body is automatic. To us it's normal, we don't think about it. When you look at it, it's wonderful how our body works. Whenever you lift your leg there is balance, which is to say muscle function. The human body is better than any autopilot built by technical means and electronics. It's so fast and precise. It's better than any machine because it's something that has been created and is part of that perfection. It's good to look at it at with a little depth because it wakes us up to see how sensational this body works. It's not just in sports, it's in day-to-day life.

Whatever we do, we need the body. Even sitting and talking you can feel the rhythm of talking and your hands moving. It's also a way of expression that's automatic. Our voice goes from very loud to very quiet through different moods. It's so precise and magic when you look at it. The more you live in the presence the more you become aware of all this functioning of your body. Autopilot is a nice description because everybody talks about it in relation to cars and planes. There is a natural autopilot within us that is much more precise. It goes to such a level of detail that it's not even visible. It would be great to be able to put this in a video and show how it functions but you really can't because the body reacts automatically, beyond vision. It's the best autopilot that has ever been made. Probably we will never be able to figure it out completely because it's so perfect that our brain is not capable of understanding. Whenever we're awake, it's always on. It's even on when we are sleeping because we keep breathing.

We should use presence more to get deeper into our body and see how it functions. It will open a lot of doors to help overcome stress and all the unpleasant feelings we have. It's like the ups and downs in our existence. We're constantly in this movement of life where it goes up and down like a wave. We fall down and we climb back up and then we fly down and sometimes it's very direct. Somehow, we always manage to get through it. If at the same time we could constantly be in the presence with the intellect functioning, we could run our mind from conscious awareness, what we really are. Then life could be something very interesting because for the time being the mind is running us. And that's where the short circuit of our humanity is.

It will probably take a while to get there, but it just shows you there is a potential, which is something to look forward to; there is a possibility, there is a way which evolution can go. It could be like the French expression where it would become *paradisiaque*—paradise. It's a good name. That's the vision we have to develop—that's the only way to go. The right way. To come to a point where we become conscious of the evolution of going in that direction and not from the head but from the heart.

Second Wind

The second wind happens when we are running out of energy and are trying very hard at whatever we do in sports or work. Then it comes to a degree where we let go and then the second wind comes in and we can go on almost endlessly.

They use that expression a lot in cross-country skiing. You come to a point of tiredness where you think you can't go on and then something happens. You let go and the rhythm kicks in. The second wind is a well-known expression in sports, because it's the rhythm. It's just a phrase we can use instead of always saying rhythm. The

Breakthrough

second wind is also a breakthrough. I like the expression "second wind" because it's not something material like wind. It's an expression and it's also an experience. It's the same as when you let go of something, you have no hang-ups. It's also in a way an autopilot. When you hike and get to a crisis point that's got you down because you have a lot farther to walk, you let go, slow down a little bit and the energy soon comes. It's like a second wind.

Even when you drive a car you can have a second wind. When you're on a trip where you have to drive 500 miles and you have only driven 100, you're already fed up and tired but you have another 400 to go. You accept it, let go and just keep going. Something kicks in and you're on your way to finding a flow where it becomes harmonious. You accept your situation and then it happens. The second wind is actually the name of another facet of the breakthrough.

I knew a mountain guide who used my approach while climbing. He was a Matterhorn guide and every day would go up to the hut where they would send the climbers from the office. He used awareness when the clients got into a situation and gave up physically and mentally because they were too tired from not getting enough oxygen; they were not used to the height. Then he would tell them to just feel the rope, feel your breathing, feel the rock and don't think about being tired. Then climbers would catch the second wind right away.

A Question of Balance

When you are on the edge of your skis, automatically your body angle wants to be in the center, to avoid falling down. Eighty percent of the falls that happen when you're skiing are against the hill because the skier is afraid of the downhill slope. It looks like you are leaning away from the mountain but actually you're not. When you let go and use your bodyweight and you're relaxed, then the body adapts automatically to the right angle of the snow. When you go too fast, you get in trouble. To hold that speed, you use your strength and then you become uptight and get tired. When you let go, you get to that place which is very subtle, where you can feel that the right quality of edging is there. Then it becomes totally effortless. Then you're floating, and it's very pleasant.

To recuperate when you're on a ski run fighting in the middle of a problem situation because it's going wrong, you automatically use some strength and your body quickly tightens up. It takes a lot of energy to fight the mistake—that happens. But when you're using your bodyweight and feeling, you don't get into that situation. You make fewer mistakes because the gravity of the body will adjust when you're relaxed. It's the natural way. It's again like walking. You adjust to the right angle by feeling. And when you walk on a path in the mountains and it's not even, it's tilted, you're on the edge of the boot on the mountainside. When you step on the other foot, you feel you're in the same balance just as you do when you're skiing. You don't think about it and you don't have to concentrate because the body has a capacity of adapting to be in perfect synchronization.

Think of a baby learning to walk. When he or she finally stands up, they are shaky; however, the baby doesn't think, but simply feels what works. There's a capability of balance in the body so we don't really have to concentrate. And when you're on a steep mountain and you're in a turn, you're on the edge and you'll feel the pressure. If at the same time you use your strength, fear comes in and then the possibility of catching an edge and falling is much greater. When you're relaxed, your body will naturally adapt.

When you ski a downhill and there's a series of bumps where it becomes really wild and right at the limit, you

The White Game

just absorb it with the skis if you're totally relaxed. It's like a car with its shock absorbers. Confidence takes effect and nothing happens, you don't catch an edge. But if you're slightly uptight the skis will cut somewhere and you'll crash. The capability of the balance of the body is much better than we can imagine. When you begin feeling the balance it means you're in total presence and there's also more joy. If you concentrate on sensing that balance it's very good for your awareness, whatever you do, like skiing, any other kind of sports or work.

When I was younger we would use a saw or a sledgehammer working in the woods; balance then becomes very important because your whole body is in motion and the body adapts all alone. All you concentrate on is the point on the piece of wood where you want to strike it. It's good to become aware and also feel the balance. You can make an exercise out of it. Just observe your body balance when you walk along the street. Now you can imagine what concentration is required for the people who walk a tightrope. Some of these crazy guys do it between two mountains and the real crazy ones do it without a safety cable. You must be out of your mind going from one point to another at that height. Not for me. I'm not willing to go that close to the edge. Life is too beautiful and precious.

Overcoming Difficulties

Overcoming difficulties is not only about being on the ski slope and having to get down at the end of a long day while supporting someone. It's also about how we do it in the real world—the slippery slopes of life.

You have a day of skiing and start out full of energy. The weather is good, the snow is perfect, everything is great and we just dance around on the skis and enjoy ourselves. Then there comes a point where we get a little tired because we can only carry on if we have a certain amount of energy. But we've lost it and need to recharge. So many times on the last run down after an incredible day I was cold and my legs hurt. My energy is gone and I'm totally empty. There's only one thing to look forward to and that's taking my skis off and walking into the ski room where at least it's warm. When you get there, you take a deep breath and relax because you made it home. When you take off your ski boots you have another a-ha experience, you feel liberated. Quite often I asked myself why the hell am I doing all this? Because when you overdo it and you're exhausted nothing makes sense anymore because we need to recuperate. We're very specialized in overdoing it, in whatever we do. We have to learn how to be reasonable. Even when you're young and go to a nightclub and dance and dance, there comes a point where you can't anymore. We seem to have great difficulty in achieving moderation.

When we're in a playing mood, in the presence and just relaxing, then we get into this harmonious state. But the goal is often excess—we always want to exaggerate instead of just cruising. I've always been amazed by the mountain guides, who really have to manage their strength because of the altitude. If you go too fast, all of a sudden you're empty, you're not going anywhere. But if you start off slowly and enjoy it, you can go on and on, all the way. The mountain guides' secret is moderation because if you're overdoing it you get tired. Top climbers will go up the north face of the Matterhorn with just crampons and spikes. Why are they doing that? You get to the top and you're completely exhausted and you made a new record and the only way you can justify it is to make an ego trip out of it. That's the only justification for your achievement: "I did it—I made a new record." Did you have fun?

I've always noticed that mountain guides, even more than instructors, are very calm people. It's because when they climb, every grip with their hands and every foot placement has to be conscious; if not, you're dead. Climbing is like meditation, it slows you down. There is a rhythm of being present, and it shows you that the breakthrough is not simply down to speed. Even in slow motion you can still be in a breakthrough experience.

There is a flow of walking, there is a flow of skiing, there's a flow of living, eating, drinking. Everybody wants to be the best, the richest, have all the power to be able to control things and other people. What for? When you get into the feeling of harmony, it doesn't make sense anymore, it really doesn't. I would like to be what an Indian teacher once said: "I am a student of life and I live in this body."

What is a Breakthrough?

A breakthrough happens when everything is in sync. When it's technically and visually 100 percent right. I can only compare it to dancing. There comes a point where your knowledge about skiing technique and style harmonizes. Then you get into the flow, which can get stronger, and at one point you start to talk about the breakthrough. Where is the breakthrough? You can't really tell because it's an experience. It's like harmoniz-

The White Game

ing with the rhythm of the music when you're dancing, letting go completely, and becoming a self-spectator. When you have beautiful music and a partner who is dancing as well as yourself at the same level, you both let go and get into the flow. That's one way of describing it. But you can't really put what a breakthrough is into words. It's a rhythm, it's a harmony, pleasure, excitement. It's a great feeling. After a breakthrough, once you stop skiing for the day you are completely ecstatic. If you're in a breakthrough there's no limit to how deep you can go. As it goes on you come to the point where it becomes ecstatic. It's an orgasm of joy.

You can even have a breakthrough experience while eating because the food tastes so good. Since dining is in the presence, in the here and now, it's real, it's not a before or after. By just sitting down and listening to good music or even when reading you get into a flow where the story becomes so fascinating, so exciting, it becomes a breakthrough. It's not only what you read, it's that you get excited physically because of the story and everything that accompanies it.

In every sport, there's the possibility of having a breakthrough. For example, in sailing when you're at the helm and you get the rhythm for how to take the waves and the noise of the wind is in your ears, everything harmonizes; you're part of the element. It's a beautiful experience. A breakthrough is harmony. That's the shortest explanation.

The breakthrough is not some huge cosmic experience but something more simple, natural, and ordinary. Not an ecstatic state where you forget your body and surroundings, but it's actually arriving at a high level. You can call it deeper or stronger but there is really no level. In certain breakthroughs, like ones I had skiing, it's also triggered by the weather, the temperature, the light in the snow when you see stars in the snow. It's harmonious. All this description is just trying to describe it, but it's a feeling. And it's a very high awareness because you become one with the surroundings and yourself—it's total presence.

The breakthrough can happen by being fully engaged in the present moment or letting go to the rhythm of your actions. We go from feeling to mindfulness, and as it grows, our identity with what we're doing fades away, and our experience becomes full awareness—that's a breakthrough. It can happen in a lot of different situations that we don't recognize at times. For example, when you go past a beautiful garden that has lovely flowers, there is this feeling. We're not aware of it but it's like a rush. Oh, it's beautiful. That's the beginning of a breakthrough. And when you're in motion, in an element like deep snow or even on a standard run, when you merge with the presence then you have a breakthrough. It can be at a very low level and it can be very strong.

Being Reasonable

When you're racing a downhill and you can feel right from the beginning when it gets rhythmic, that this is good and you control it, you trust the feeling. And without being conscious of it you try to make it even stronger. You let go, just stick to that line you have studied before and it's like an afterburner—it kicks in. You have a top performance even though the possibility that you crash is always there. When you're in that euphoric state of the breakthrough the capacity goes to the limit of 100 percent—but don't go over it. It's quite difficult to control and the racers always talk about the limit. Then there are places where you know OK, I can carve this completely with 100 percent capability. It works but it can also produce a fall. Whatever you do be reasonable. Don't exaggerate. Accept being reasonable and being sensible. Relax. Not wanting more and more. It's the want for more that's very destructive. If you're reasonable then it also becomes flawless and then you enjoy it.

It's like a skier who knows how to ski well and has perfect conditions—instead of attacking, you just enjoy it, the beautiful snow, the scenery. Instead of being aggressive, dance with it, enjoy it. It's the same thing in day-to-day life. When you experience that something functions which will make you more money, just relax and observe, don't run after more money and power. It's difficult because we are so success-oriented. Be reasonable. Find a pace in life that is comfortable.

It's like this legendary mountain guide Ulrich Inderbinen who was already over ninety when he was stationed at the hut on the Monte Rosa glacier above Zermatt. They sent a client from the guides office up to the hut to climb with him. Ulrich was forty years older than the client and when the client got to the hut he was totally shocked. He picked up his phone, called the office and said that he'd asked for a mountain guide, not a grandfather. They told him not to worry, it's not a difficult mountain, it's for people in average condition. Just listen to him and you'll be OK. He accepted that but

The White Game

he wasn't happy about it. They started out and you don't have to explain a lot because you're walking through snow that's slightly uphill, zigzagging between crevasses. The client managed to get to the top and when they got down Ulrich stayed in the hut because he had another client the next day. The client came down to the guides' office and said they were right, but next time he wanted a guide who let him stop on and off to catch his breath because Ulrich never stopped. Ulrich was never in a hurry. I've never seen him in a hurry walking down the street. He always had the same rhythm.

The key is learning to be reasonable in what we do. We have completely lost our natural rhythm. Everything is speed, speed, speed, and more and more and more. The result of it is obvious. We have accumulated and made fantastic things but at what price? The secret is an easy, reasonable life. Not to have many expectations and be present, to play. Who invented the theory that you can't play anymore when you're an adult? We all have to be serious and dressed in a certain outfit and walk in a special way. Why not take it easy even if you don't see the whole tree, only the bottom. It's still nice. It's simple except when you dream about being on the other side of the world. When I look at myself, I'm playing the same crazy game as everybody else. We're all conditioned, we've created the condition and we pay for it. We have all the comfort of everything we've accumulated but we can only do so much so we get stressed and discontented. That's why all these mountain guides are quiet. They have the rhythm. They know they can't go too fast because they will never make it to the top. They have the big picture with the whole journey in mind. And that's what makes a guide a guide. You can guide somebody, you can't really teach them, they have to do it themselves.

Both Sides of a Breakthrough

As a good skier you know when you're in the comfort zone—it feels good. You're floating, it's nice, it's pleasant. It takes a little more speed and then it gets closer to a breakthrough. At the same time, if you are fearless, you feel you can let go. Then the body takes over because you know how to ski well and you just enjoy the breakthrough. Once you're in that rhythm you can still push yourself but you have to know where your limit is. It should be as close as possible to the limit because when you watch a ski race, especially the downhill, you can see this skier is really at his limit. It doesn't mean he's got more rhythm and there might be someone else whose limit is higher than theirs. This is their best. It's the same for an intermediate skier to progressively go closer to their limit and still control and enjoy it. We love to go over our limits—it's somehow exciting but it's also dangerous.

Having a breakthrough is also a matter of understanding the bad experiences and managing them. The more we concentrate on what we're feeling, the more we see that unpleasant sensations have a certain quality, but it's no longer that black thing that ruins everything and makes us stiff and incapable and wrecks our confidence. It has its own flow, its own purpose. Looking at it from a deep place within, you become more responsible and understanding. It's the best place to be where you can accept the good and the bad and eventually you're glad the uncomfortable parts are there too. It's like a safety belt and then it becomes harmonious. You can accept both sides and not just put one on the side as the bad ghost which destroys everything. It takes on another dimension and at the same time it takes another shape the way you look at it and try to handle it.

You accept the difficulty and that it has its purpose to be there. You need enough experience to be able to look at it from a place where it becomes clear what its value is. Maybe it's even at a point where that thing also becomes harmonious. It's part of us and it's not just the black devil; it's my partner. It's part of the total structure. You have to accept everybody on the team because we're definitely not alone in this body; there are a lot of obstacles and things going on but they all have their purpose. It has to become harmonious. Accept all these different things and then you can really grow and enjoy it because you have accepted the good and bad. It's beautiful.

Flatland Breakthrough

There is always the possibility of finding a breakthrough outside of sports. It's the effect of totally letting go and trusting your know-how of what you're doing and then your actions become very rhythmic. Then it flows and there's a breakthrough.

People can have a breakthrough by, for example, writing a book or short stories, and when they're finished there is a sense of harmony and it feels complete. There's a satisfied feeling of "that's it." The satisfaction is also a breakthrough. When I started talking about the breakthrough it was just through describing speed or balance or something like that but the breakthrough is much bigger. It exists on every level of life. Reading a book will also produce that breakthrough because everything we do has that potential. When we start learning how to swim, all of a sudden it works. It clicks. It's like when you trust your balance riding a bicycle. You're in motion, up on that edge and have movement, complete balance because you are in motion.

While in a meeting in the business world you can practice your listening skills to be aware. Focused listening when someone's talking brings you into your presence. And if somebody interrupts the dialogue while you're in a meeting, instead of staying with your aggravation you really listen. Then because the listening makes you present, you start getting into the conversation. But if you listen to your frustrated mind trying to say you shouldn't have come here, this is all a waste of time or whatever the mind says, then it's very difficult to be present. We have to listen and sometimes I'm so absent I don't even notice what's being said. And then other times I'm right there and then it's full of joy. It can be applied to everything. Try to live more in the presence than in your head and then things will work. That's the secret.

The Mind

The mind will analyze everything and hinder you from doing your best work or having the most engagement possible in a meeting. The mind is very vicious because it will mislead you. In business, you can make a big thing out of a problem and almost get into a depression. Then again, if you have some experience in letting go, if you can catch your mental activity at that moment and move on, then you start to control it. That's definitely the best tool we have. There is no doubt about it and it doesn't need a pill and it doesn't need some kind of medicine. To learn how to let go, you have to concentrate on something that's always there and it's the breath. It's above and beyond explanations of what it is. It's that life energy.

Focus

When I go hiking and I'm thinking with my dreaming mind, I don't enjoy it. To remedy this, from the beginning I listen to whatever is there, like the wind, or else focus on what I see—vision is very powerful. When you walk and you look at nature, the flowers, the trees, the valley, the mountains, it somehow produces presence. Then you get into the flow very easily. And once you're in that flow of enjoyment, of hiking and at the same time feeling the surroundings, then you're happy, you appreciate it.

You also go much further than you planned to because you enjoy it and you're in a flow. From the flow, it takes very little to get to where it becomes what you could call ecstatic, and then you're in the breakthrough. Even on an intellectual level, when you're interested enough, you let go to the subject you're studying, get into the flow and also enjoy it. There is the presence—it's the secret of joy.

People are really touched when they have a breakthrough. Some make statements like "that was sensational" or "that was out of this world." What they feel is their experience. You can tell because they're glowing, they look happy. You can see there's a great satisfaction of contentment. You might even call it fulfillment. The possibility exists of developing, going deeper into an experience where it's even more beautiful. Even though I'm getting older and my skiing gets slower, on the outside I still glow. That's the miracle.

Break on Through

It's important to make clear that a breakthrough is not

Breakthrough

just a goal. The breakthrough begins already by feeling comfortable when you slide, walking on the skis, feeling the poles and the balance. It's a buildup. When there is a certain amount of knowledge, of experience, you reach that point where it becomes ecstatic. The breakthrough begins to grow. It happens alone—we don't make the breakthrough. It's the whole knowledge, understanding, and the practicing. Then the joy will come to a point where it flips and you become a spectator full of joy.

Once it starts to work, when a novice student manages to start changing directions, they have this feeling of "I'm starting to control that." It's a fulfilling feeling at a very low level but that's how a breakthrough starts and then it will grow. The breakthrough will happen on its own when you practice the simple exercises of feeling but you cannot make it a goal. Breakthrough is a great sensation, not just in skiing but in everything you do. It's an effect of the whole learning process and then it'll come the point where the joy just turns over and it becomes a real game.

I was always fascinated by this thing called nirvana. It's part of that simplicity, the inner self. When people read that word, they imagine being in a heaven of this totality, but it's not real. It's a dream. But when you experience this calm, when you become really still, you start to feel that harmony. It starts to feel a little bit like when you begin to sleep but you don't go to sleep. It's outrageous to hear that definition because it doesn't fit at all the concept of nirvana, samadhi, or anything like that. Fulfillment—you can't draw it—it's a pure feeling. Trying to explain simplicity makes it too complicated to understand with our thinking brain. For a little kid who's in the presence, it's natural and clear. That's what it is—contentment, joy, fulfillment. Somehow your body awareness is gone and all you feel is that floating feeling.

The basic thing is not to aim for reaching a point where you go into nirvana and then, afterward, go into samadhi. It's an imagination and has absolutely no reality while the true reality is unbelievably simple. It also has its purity. When you look at a child who doesn't even walk or talk or anything—it just looks at you with these eyes—the look is so outrageous. It speaks more than any words. You can feel it with your heart if you know what's going on. It doesn't need any explanation. A breakthrough is like growing a potato. I have to say something stupid to lighten up this subject! What we experience in the presence is much more real than any name like nirvana or samadhi. It's that feeling. Beyond

Breakthrough

the physical part, it's beyond words or anything. You can't really explain it but you can feel it, whether you're uneducated or a genius.

A breakthrough is not some kind of a goal-oriented exercise. It's an evolution, an experience. Truth is very simple. It's not some kind of ultimate realization or explosion into the light.

Visualization

What is Visualization?

Visualization exists in every activity we do. It's already happening spontaneously in the lives of every child. A child learns to walk by imitating the grown-ups. When we're kids and don't even know how to walk, we get up on our knees and watch an older child. They're already standing and we observe them, imitate them, and stand up. We might fall down again but eventually, we will find the center of balance, and then we're standing. When children are introduced to gymnastics or skiing it's the same thing—they visualize.

We use visualization throughout our whole life. It's a very important aspect as it's part of the awareness we experience via our senses. Visualization is the greatest way to learn. When we do sports as kids we look at the good skiers, and even when we're adults we also look at the better skiers and want to ski like them. We imitate

Visualization

and sometimes it feels harmonious. At first, it might feel awkward, but then after you have practiced it for some time you have a breakthrough. When you practice something, you will discover your flow. At a very low level it becomes fluid, it becomes easy and you start to fly.

Visualization goes 100 percent through life, even if you become a fighter pilot. In a flight simulator they show you the right and the wrong things and you can actually visualize it. Visualization teaches you what to do and what not to do. Whatever sports you do, you're always imitating the ones who have achieved the feeling of a breakthrough, of knowing. Even on an intellectual level it's like another dimension and when you learn something new like a language there is also imitation.

Theory is good but you follow it with an action and then it becomes experience. It's very clear that the theory has vanished because it became experience, being present. You don't need the theory anymore because what we have is feeling and in the feeling is joy, knowing, harmony. It's like curiosity—you think about an action but when you feel it then it becomes real. Thinking about it is part of the process, a communication of feeling.

The White Game
If You Can See It, You Can Do It

There are three steps in learning to race by imitating the top skiers: first, come to a point where you feel you're 100 percent copying them. Then, get to where you're performing well. Finally, visualize your own breakthrough and go beyond.

When I saw big champions skiing a certain sequence, I imitated that image and very quickly got the hang of it. I would watch them carefully and when I skied in races I saw the skier in my imagination and I copied them. The interesting thing is you come to a point where you make progress. You discover there's a great rhythm, like dancing. And the more you let go, the deeper you go into the presence, which is where the awareness kicks in. We call it the breakthrough. You can feel that the copy is right and there comes a point where you imitate your own breakthrough. That's how you progress.

I only used visualization to learn and progress. All the top racers do it like that because imitating the best ones is a very powerful learning technique. When you get to the point where the copy is working, you can feel it. It's not a theory, it's an experience. Once you knew you could do it when you were training, you were able to get into the rhythm right away in a race because it's

Visualization

a feeling.

Another example is when you visualize going on a downhill run. You go through the course in your mind and you can even feel it—the speed, the pressure, and the bumps. In a race, the visualization starts about five minutes before your turn to go. You get excited and then at the last minute, it's almost euphoric. You push off and you're in the race. You'd better be in the here and now because otherwise, you're not going to go far before crashing.

You have to be as relaxed as possible in a race. If there is any tension in your body you've had it, there's no way of winning. When you get into a perfect flow really early and find the line then it's a breakthrough run and you feel it when it's perfect. You have to get into the rhythm right from the beginning, and once you are in it then it can become even stronger. The stronger it gets the more you let go because you know you are on the plan and that's the way you wanted to do it. You feel that it's the best you've done, all the way to the finish and you can win.

Whenever I've won, all I wanted was to race faster than anybody else. I did everything I knew to make it fast and it all clicked together. And before they announced it on the loudspeaker, I knew this was it, even if I came in second or third. If I placed after that I had my excuses: I didn't have the right angle on one turn, too much edging, not enough letting go. There's lots of things to blame, lots of excuses. You feel it when it's an excellent result. It's more like it's a top performance for yourself. It doesn't really have anything to do with winning. You know you gave your best and it was good because you judge yourself. You recognize when you are in sync and where everything went according to the plan.

If you're in a total breakthrough from the beginning to the end, then you're not even surprised when they announce your best time. You knew it was good.

It would be an obstacle to visualize that you're going to win. When you do that, if it's just a vision, you will not win, it's not real. I've never had a vision of winning. I wanted to win but I didn't have an image of it.

Visualization—See it to Feel It

On the ski run, you always see good skiers and crazy skiers. Then there are the exceptions, such as a person who really has style and looks harmonious. They look like they're dancing on the snow. You get very interested and if you're free and not with a class you can follow

Visualization

them at a certain distance. There are challenging sections this great skier skis and you observe how they do it. Afterward, when you are alone and visualize the person skiing in your mind's eye, as realistically as when you were watching them, that's where you try to emulate them. That's how imitating really happens.

You can feel it when you start doing it the same way. You have that vision and then you practice it. You might feel you haven't got it yet but you keep doing it and then all of a sudden you notice you have a sort of breakthrough. You know from the feeling that you now have this graceful way of turning, letting go completely to the rhythm and you practice it. To imitate it you have to find a place which is similar to where you saw the person skiing because that goes hand-in-hand. You can even go to the same place. Once you have the image and you know you can do it as well as the image, it becomes your own property.

You can let go of the image but you can always go back and check if you still have it in your head. If you're not there every day, your mind will tell you that you can't do it anymore. Then you have to practice and you'll know when you've got it again. It's like pulling out a drawer and taking the image out again and imitating it. You can feel it when you're there, it's a sort of game.

Inner Learning

We can even learn by practicing presence. It's a certain visualization too. You look deep within yourself and you reach a place of profound stillness with a sense of timeless peace. Being in the present moment will open up your heart and soul. You learn that by practicing, not just listening to people talk about it. If you get turned on by listening about living in the now, then try it out yourself. Maybe a whole lot more than you ever imagined will open up for you. And that's called knowledge of the self.

Even if you have a disability you still have your inner self. You can go there and find a rhythm and a breakthrough. I see a possibility even for people with disabilities to go to a place which is not a physical level—just consciousness. And because of their disability, they'll go even deeper because they are not in competition on a physical level (unless they're a Paralympian). As far as the feeling goes you don't need to talk, all you have to do is feel that inner self. Even if they can't express it, it still makes them happy. There is a huge potential.

VISUALIZATION
Changing a Bad Mood to Good

You can also visualize yourself out of a bad mood. If you're capable of visualizing it, then you already start becoming conscious that you're in one.

You don't really want to be in a bad mood and by becoming aware of the negative pattern you want to get rid of it. The more you experience it consciously, the more you will start letting go of it. You know it's just a concept but if you give into being in a bad mood then you're lost. The more you practice being aware of it, the more you let go of it.

It's like practicing awareness, whatever your discipline. You'll notice that when you look at it you have already pushed it a little bit to the side and you can look at it objectively. But when that negative state of mind possesses you, you're lost. There's not much you can do about it and you don't even want to do anything, you just want to be in a bad mood.

The more you look at it, the more you'll control it and let it go. By that letting go, it puts us in a state where we can look at things from a detached perspective. When we're in the concept and identify with "I'm a moody person," what are you going to do? You just have to live it out, go

The White Game

and have a drink or swear or whatever. But when you look at it and just stand there, there's a separation. Then when you practice that awareness, you get stronger. It becomes clear: I'm moody and I don't want to be moody anymore. You look at it and distance yourself further until finally you control it.

When you're in a bad mood you can tell yourself "here comes my mind again. It's trying to drive me crazy but I'm not for hire." Really show it that the bad mood is not you and you don't want anything to do with it. That's the fantastic thing about being present and letting go. It puts everything aside. That's why it's called letting go. To be in a place where there's nothing else but the sound of your breath, what you hear, what you feel, what you say, and just groove on that. It's where that creative energy comes from and it's not words anymore. We finally reach a place where we can see very clearly. You're in the experience of the presence and that's positive—which is another name.

We have a name for everything. We are very good intellectuals, philosophical thinkers, and all that, but it's either you feel or you think. If you want to be with your thinking and give all your rights to your mind, then you've had it. If we want to have a good experience

Visualization

and be relaxed and enjoy it then we practice presence. It relaxes us and out of the relaxation comes joy, all the way to love. Which is again another name, a top name. It's really a feeling, a letting go. It doesn't need any names.

Managing Fear

Nature of Fear

Fear can come from being in extreme nature, competition, danger, injuries, and failure. Physical fear is panic. When I was racing there was a certain nervousness before the race started. I don't know whether it was fear or just tension because the atmosphere in a race is something more than everyday relaxed skiing. But as soon as you're out of the starting gate and get to the feeling of the mountain then the fear is gone, because if not, you won't go very far—you'll crash.

Fear is there. It does its thing—it comes from the mind. In truth, it's an illusion because the mind doesn't want to let go since it likes to always control us. We've been brainwashed and given all the authority to the mind and it runs us. The only thing I can say is fear, OK, it's there. Let it do its thing but don't go for it. Just let it go by like a cloud and concentrate on breathing.

Managing Fear

To overcome fear, feel the present moment—wherever you are or whatever you're doing. Whether it's sports or work or some other activity. Whatever we do is the chance to be present. When we're living in the moment we let go because inside we know what we're doing. When we think too much, we don't know what we're doing. Being aware takes away fear. When I watch people learn, learning to trust themselves, the expression on their face changes from fear to elation.

Fear is an illusion; a dream that possesses us because somehow, it's part of us. It also has a point where it becomes positive because it keeps us from skiing over our heads and getting hurt. Just let it run and don't even think about how you're going to stop it. It's there, so accept it and take that little thing of positivity and put it into the total experience. Then once you feel that what you're doing works, that you can handle it, the fear is gone. It's replaced by euphoria and joy.

Without anyone telling you, you can actually see when a student is experiencing fear. The person is all stiff. Even when they're only standing still; you tell them to let go, don't worry, nothing bad will happen. Just be at ease like when you have no skis on. Relax and feel the snow and the edging. Right away when they start letting go they become quite confident.

My job as a teacher is to really put myself into the situation of what the student is going through because I know from experience the emotions they are feeling. All I have to do is see what can I do so the student can loosen up.

Fear also has an exciting aspect. It's this wonder and the big question: can I do it? It's a sort of doubting, but when you experience you can do it, it's canceled. It goes back to being a dream or an illusion. It doesn't exist whatever it is. Fear also has a positive aspect for protection. This can be experienced in the traffic during high season on a ski run where there are a lot of people and everybody's racing. And it gets wild. Especially in the late afternoon after they've had lunch, a lot to drink, and smoked a joint—they become totally careless. They're completely out of their heads and they don't see the danger. They don't care, there's no respect—it's dangerous. It's safer to race because there's nobody in the way. You have 20 meters on each side to crash and slow down and if you don't stop at the end the nets will do the rest.

Beyond Fear

When grown-ups start to learn skiing, they are quite

Managing Fear

stiff because there is tension everywhere and they're not sure of themselves and lack belief. But as soon as they see something that works in what they're doing, the fear goes away. When trust comes in it tells you, OK, I can do this, I can control it. Then the joy comes even more and that's where you're starting to have the breakthrough. You really go for it and you're in that state of an out-of-body experience. You fly and you control it. When there is no fear and tension in your body then you let go totally to the state of being present. You break through and there's nothing bad that can happen. You can always hit a bump that throws you off balance and could cause a crash but you don't think about that. You don't have the time because you're too busy enjoying the breakthrough. Fear is an illusion. Fear is not knowing, that's all. But when you know, the fear goes away.

When you have fear and are insecure, you're totally in your mind. It's only when you go to the present moment and feel something in the state of presence that it starts to go away. It tells you: it's OK, I can handle it. That's why it's so important to be present and feel what you do and not think about it. We need to think in order to function but we only control something when at the same time we are experiencing it. Otherwise you just

The White Game

stay stiff and dislike whatever you're doing. When you're starting out as a skier and not sure about what you're doing and full of fear, you can't get into it because you're totally in your mind. You're a prisoner of your mind and it's not a very pleasant experience. It always comes back to the same thing. Do something that brings you back to the presence. Then things function. I experience that it works, but sometimes it's very difficult to put into words because it's so simple. When you get in that state of spontaneity, then the joy is there too. When I refer to what I'm feeling when I ski, then all the negative stuff disappears, I fly, I glide.

I was listening to an interview, the other day, with an old man in America who was a good friend of the Dalai Lama. He said the Dalai Lama was present more or less all the time. I really enjoyed hearing that because that's the secret. It's true, whenever I've seen some film of the Dalai Lama, he looks like he is extremely relaxed. That's the only way I can explain it. He somehow shines, he glows, because at the same time there is no structure, no tension, no figuring out—it's just being. Like the words of Shakespeare: "To be or not to be?" Or maybe The Beatles: "Let it be."

Managing Fear

Moving on from Fear

As a teacher, I have to know what the student can or can't do. I have to be careful not to take too much risk but then also not step back too much. I have to adapt to their knowledge level before I take them on a black run. I completely concentrate on what they're doing when we begin. We start off slowly so they can get confident about being able to handle the route. When you observe them right at the beginning you can find out if it's too early to be trying. When that has happened I have canceled the approach. I put it off for later and we go down a red run instead of a black one.

I tell them if they feel stiff and notice fear or some kind of nervousness, stand still—breathe. Let go and relax—that's the first step. Then we will start out slowly to observe what they're feeling. I tell them to feel the contact with the snow, do the turns slowly, and relax. Usually, they calm down, loosen up a little bit. If they haven't fallen after one or two turns they get more confident right away; yes, I can do it even if it's very shaky. I have gone around the complete turn. Everything is fine, so the confidence comes in. Maybe on the second turn it's half-and-half, but then it works again and gives them more confidence. A little more fear and stiffness goes away and eventually they get into a slow flow. Confidence also comes and it makes the student secure and trusting. The confidence comes up when that know-how is there in the feeling. Every turn will be another success and will become better, more solid.

The more you let go, the more flawless it gets. Finally, you come to a state where you feel the capability of "I can do this." That will help you in letting go even more and then you trust it. The more confidence you have, the smoother it gets and the better you turn. Then it comes to a point where at the end of the run the student is blissed out because now they have the confirmation: I can make that step to the black run, which means I can ski everywhere.

That's how you work on fear so the student builds confidence. They know that if they take it easy and are relaxed they can do it without too much speed and not get quickly out of control. A fall is always a possibility, but when they're going slowly, not skiing over their limit, the body reacts automatically and will correct itself. When you're skiing beyond your ability, that's when you lose control. Then it becomes a hazard. We have so many years of experience of walking, we don't even think about it. There are usually no problems but

Managing Fear

sometimes we trip because we are not conscious of what we're walking on. We have to be conscious of what we're doing.

If you are a fearless person, you like stepping on the gas, you like speed. Then when you crash, the level of fear is back up at the top again. Then it's more difficult for the student to let go, but when they go slowly they feel that it works.

A teacher has to constantly analyze the student and observe what they're doing, how well they are doing, how stiff they are, whether they look relaxed. By being calm they can sometimes get spaced out and absent-minded but they still have to feel the contact with the snow to be present. When you have that connection, that awareness of the client, it also gives you a lot of confidence. You learn and you grow with it on another level, the level of understanding, caring. There's nothing to be proud of—it's more a thankfulness of being able to get to the depths where somebody is not physically hooked up to you.

I've heard so many stories from mountain guides. If their students don't have the rope hooked into their harness, clipped in, they are completely stiff. I've heard from guides that some people literally shiver because the fear is really shaking them. And as soon as they are clipped in and the rope is not pulled but snug then it's gone—they let go, they feel safe. Giving the client that security is one of the most important things in climbing. They're not just hooked up by the rope, they're also mentally secure. When a guide is in the summer trek traffic and takes somebody up the Matterhorn and down again, everything can work well and function without interference, but there are always little things that can go wrong. When they materialize, they happen very quickly and a lot of the climbers say thank you when they're back at the hut.

Mountains are mountains, they are powerful. It's beautiful to be in their company and respect fear and play with that experience. It's beautiful. Because fear is there, it's real. Even though I say it doesn't exist, it's part of an illusion because the mind supports it and says yes. The more you listen to it the stiffer you get. It's part of the game. Life in general is like that. It's not something else, it's all part of life.

Adrenaline Rush

My friend Sylvain Saudan the early extreme skier was interviewed once with two champion extreme skiers

Managing Fear

and was asked: "What do you think about how it's developed?" He answered: "After 30 or 40 meters I would stop and look around and enjoy it. And these guys today are in a panic, afraid." He also said: "It's very interesting to live close to the red line, but you know you can't take the step over it." Being a thrill seeker keeps you sharp and creates a heightened awareness and this level of intensity definitely requires being present.

I haven't done extreme skiing but when I hear somebody like Sylvain talk about it I get an impression of what the intensity of that experience is. His statement was that "when I look at them and the way they do it and the time they do it in, the descent of 1000 meters in 15 or 20 seconds can only be in total fear and panic and hope that you will survive." They translated it into a kick, an incredible experience. It's lucky that they get to the bottom alive. I cannot imagine what it really feels like.

You have to just let it run because it's so fast, with the huge jumps you take over cliffs, landing in very steep deep snow where you have nothing solid to slow you down. It can only be what he called a total panic. I guess people can have a breakthrough experience in those situations. At a very high level they probably do because after they've done it two or three times and nothing has

The White Game

happened, it gives them confidence. Each time you do it, you're at the maximum of the limit and there it's another limit of not just crashing. It's life and death because when you fall and happen to land on the rocks with your shoulders and neck—you've had it. There's not one bone in their body that will not break because of the speed they're going and the power they develop.

There is fear and there is an elation after they stop. This is also the release of the fear because they made it alive, they were playing with death. It's going very far to play with your existence to that extent. You've got to be a little crazy. When you do it the way the first guys did it, like Sylvain and Reinhold Messner, they were doing it at a speed where they could control it and even have some fun, feeling comfortable, safe, and not in a panic.

It looks very attractive when you see movies that put a positive spin on it, and it inspires young crazy kids to do the same thing. However, it puts them in danger with no respect for their existence but they do it just for kicks.

I don't believe that there is no fear. To me, it's not possible. Everybody has that source of fear in them even though they are the best at what they do. It's interesting to go to the lengths of putting myself into this situation

Managing Fear

because I can imagine what it feels like to jump off a ledge into a hill and with the first landing, already half the slope is starting to move as an avalanche. You start to ski in that fast-moving snow and the next thing is a cliff where you fly 50 to 60 meters through the air. You don't even know if where you land there are sharp rocks 20 centimeters under the snow. Mountains are made of rocks and when you hit one you have no chance, you're gone. And to say it's not fear, it's a kick—to me they're lying to themselves.

The need for speed is like driving a car fast—it's a rush. I know that rush because I've been racing where you ski a steep run at 120 or 130 kilometers an hour or even more. It can reach 135 or even 140 in Kitzbühel, Austria. There you have to concentrate very hard. You've got to be right in the moment because if not, you've had it. When you lose control at that speed you don't know what's going to happen—you're going to crash. And sometimes the crashes are even scary to look at.

The racers feel the adrenaline but they control it. They have physical training, but you as a normal skier can't go down the hill like a racer because you're not in the same condition. It's dangerous for you and everyone else on the run.

The White Game

Feeling Fear

The worst fear is the fear of fear. That's what we all worry about. Why focus on fear? It's not going to solve anything. We're afraid that we're going to fall and break a leg, end up in the hospital, won't be able to run our business, and all that. The risk is there. You can ski down or you can take the cable car. And then the cable car can fall while all the skiers are having fun on the slope.

Fear is a terrible thing—we all have it to a certain extent. When we can look at fear instead of experiencing fear we can laugh about it. When it's there and we don't laugh about it that's because we are in the state where it dominates us. When we have fear and then experience something that works, then right away we don't even remember we were afraid—it's just gone. It's like it never existed because we're in control.

The Moment Called Now

Being Present

When I'm with a client up on the mountain and they put on the skis, I tell them to just look all around at the different peaks. Notice what the temperature is, what the weather's like, whether there's wind, and notice the intensity of the light in the snow. I make them aware of where they are and the elements. Then I say look at how the skiers are zooming around. Once they are really present, we start the ski lesson. It's very important to do that, so before they even ski, they become aware of where they are.

When you're present in whatever you do, you're energized. But when you're totally in your mind, your recharging system is blocked. You're not renewing energy, you're only spending energy. You very quickly become frustrated and stressed. When you're present there's harmony happening which is constantly ener-

The White Game

gizing and you feel good, it's pleasant. It's like listening to music that we like, which we think is harmonious, we let go and listen and are in the presence. When we listen we very quickly come to a point where we stand up and dance to it because there is joy. Being present means being joyous. It's actually very simple. Even when we eat, when there is good food, we feel that joy, we feel that satisfaction. We know we need food to strengthen our physical system. But it also feeds our heart, our true being, our contentment, and our happiness.

If we're constantly figuring out with the mind what we can do to make ourselves richer or more powerful, we're really going in the direction of feeding the ego and going down the wrong path. That's why this expression is interesting—to be or not to be. When we're in that power game and have that longing for wealth and influence, we're on the wrong track. We prefer good food, to dance, to ski or swim or whatever it is that is pleasant for us. Being present is pleasant. We are completely blind when we're trying to figure out how we can make more money and have more power. When we look around, those things haven't made us happy. Even those who have them, they still like to eat, they still like to sleep, play, love, to listen to some kind of good music or see a

The Moment Called Now

beautiful view of nature.

The presence is all around us. It's with every breath—that's why conscious breathing is so pleasant. When we are under stress and all of a sudden we take that deep breath, even if it's just a fraction of a second of presence, the energy comes in and gives us a certain balance and equilibrium again. We go on until we have to take the next deep breath and be conscious again for a split second, to be in the moment.

When somebody eats delicious food and says "that was good," you look in their eyes and see that it's good. Even that look makes us feel good. And if you eat the same thing, you have the same feeling from the taste of that food. It's joy because it's harmony, like seeing a spectacular sunset. That's the presence, that's heaven. We have to practice that heaven. Everybody should know it and talk about it, be clear and have a conscious experience of that positive side—not the intoxication of power and money. Everybody says we need money to live and to have authority to control things. What are we controlling? In truth when you go deeper into the presence you start to notice that we're not controlling anything, it's controlling us. It's giving us this contentment and peace. That's presence.

The White Game

Vision

We imitate through our whole life and even at my age, I'm visualizing. One day I was at the top of the valley surrounded by these beautiful mountains. Admiring this beautiful creation, I had this feeling deep down that felt harmonious, creative and at the same time, I saw that we always want to make things better. They say at the end of your life you go downhill but that's not true. You still have this life force that makes you want to enjoy your existence. For our inner self to notice this there's only one thing to do to get to that point which is to practice presence. It's possible in whatever we do—driving, dancing, eating, traveling. By practicing this, you get into a feeling of harmony where you see that everything that's alive is hooked up.

Your life is something in perfect balance otherwise you wouldn't be living. That's the quality of life. To get to that depth you have to live in the moment because until now we've only gone in one direction and that's our mind. There's another dimension and that's going inward. It intensifies your feelings, and when you feel something good, it becomes very good. It also makes you appreciate. The next thing is conscious thankfulness and that's when you are at the door of the inner breakthrough.

The Moment Called Now

We all visualize but visualization can be envisioning problems, which would lead us to live in a world of problems. When we're dreaming of good things and we look at our mind, within part of the mind negative stuff comes in. But your vision can be something more elevated, you can have a visualization as a guiding light, a principal. We can have a vision of beauty and beautiful things and the aggression is always pushed aside because we like that beauty more. The deeper we go into the experience, the better it gets. The more we do it, the less space there is for the negative things. Letting go to what we feel, not what we think because a lot of the thinking stuff doesn't bring us anything. Feeling will make our awareness grow and the more we enjoy it, the more we will practice it. Eventually, we come to a place where maybe there will be harmony not just for us, but our whole world. Because it's for everybody.

How Being Present Creates a Personal Vision

When you practice presence, you increase the intensity of how you look at things. When you see a beautiful vista or a scenic ocean there comes a moment where automatically the feeling comes up of how incredible creation really is and how it has been created by some kind of divine energy. You become clear that there must be a power that has created this. A creative energy, because it's there, I live it, see it, hear it, feel it and even taste it. Then the heart starts to wake up. That's when it speaks—when you see the beauty, when you see that divine creation. That power lives, it's alive. Everything is alive, even the mountains. It took the Matterhorn eons to travel from Africa to the Alps. At that time, we didn't have countries, we didn't have a name for the creation, but it was there. Always was and always will be.

We've gone very far in the universe and we're only scratching the surface and getting a little taste of eternity. That again is creation. We can feel the power of infinite energy. It's in the form of the joy of a beautiful view, of beautiful people who can see it, can speak it, who glow, even not saying anything, because they practice presence. Our heart cries out for it. We need it and yet we already have it. That's why it comes down to the very simple thing—when we were born all we had was contentment. When something was desired, the basic need of food, then we were happy because that's all we needed and now we want lots of things. But the essential thing is the lasting one.

The most thankful moment is when we have the depth

The Moment Called Now

to see and experience the creator of the energy because when I look at you, and everybody else, we're all breathing the same stuff. We all have that capacity to actually see God, feel it in our hearts, and know that it's the source of that energy. We don't have to look for God—his omnipresence gives us life; it gives us everything.

It's not complicated, it's always the same thing: practicing being conscious. Practicing being human. We have to. We have to restart the humanization. It's like everything we do, the more we practice, the better we get. But then someone says "the music is beautiful and good food is wonderful but I have to work." And at the same time, there is a certain aggravation because it takes a lot of effort. Do you really have to work that much or can work become secondary and the joy come first? When we were born and had nothing, all we had was joy.

Because of the constraints of our social system and the way we work, we need to develop the art of being present so we can enjoy life. It makes sense to earn money so we have enough to live. Everything has become so exaggerated that most people say I don't have time for such secondary things. They forgot completely that it's the most important thing. If we don't have our breath, we don't have anything. We can't make money, we can't control anything—which we don't anyway, it's just a concept. By controlling things what do we gain?

War is the biggest game and the money that's made behind it. All our so-called civilized countries produce these incredible weapons and sell them to the governments who are making wars against us. Where is the sense? It doesn't make sense anymore. Everybody is selling arms and they finally get into the hands of the terrorists and it backfires on us. Most people even know this but just ignore it. The mind pushes it away because the money businesses make out of it is so overriding and important that it hides the truth. Instead of working together and enjoying life, one country wants to be better than the other. Better than what? We breathe the same air, we live on the same planet. At the moment it doesn't make sense anymore. That's probably because we're in the middle of the Kali Yuga, the dark age, as described in Indian literature.

That's why the solution is so simple—to practice presence. It doesn't need money, you don't have to buy it, you don't have to pay for it. What you get from it is everything. You get clarity, understanding, and joy. You see what is dark and what is light. Our denomination is **power and wealth**. Everybody says that's the system.

The Moment Called Now

But systems can change and they do constantly. That's why we have to practice living in the moment. It's so easy to sit down and listen to your breath because it relaxes you. You can do it any place and at any time. That's where your heart is.

When we say heart, the average person sees the muscle that pumps the blood, that's all and we know it's very important. It's also scary for some people to even think about their life. It lasts so many years even though it's just a twinkle of existence. That it exists is a miracle—but we don't see life as a miracle. We think life is there to become rich and powerful. The other heart hasn't got a label or menu like materialism. That heart is free. It's also free of religion, free of philosophy. The only thing it has is feeling. We have to understand what feeling really is because if you want to know God then you have to practice awareness. If we ignore that and are just interested in accumulating material things, the energy we have to invest to reach that is not very rewarding. Look at all these businessmen running around like crazy, stressed out and taking pills all the time just to be able to function, even to sleep. When you become aware of that power, you can always plug into it, feeling that it's breathing you—that's it. It really comes to that point where you can't even talk about it, you cannot express it anymore, it's beyond words. It's just feeling happiness, clarity, and contentment. And the source of it is—life.

Developing a Personal Vision

Peacefulness is when you feel peace, freedom and that everything is fine. Contentment. You're happy, whatever you do. You have accepted everything. And since you know that there is an endless part of you, a form of energy, you can sit down and enjoy it. When you're feeling good you've realized something to get to this stage of contentment. When you experience it then you also know there is no end to it. You can also practice being at peace more to be happier and get closer to heaven. What else is there to do? To have only one desire to go deeper. Being in the now helps you in developing individual character, style, and learning to live your life in a more positive way. These are guiding principles that lead to us having a better-quality life and it gets better the more you practice it.

There's a breakthrough on the physical level and there's one on the mental level that includes your outlook of life, the purpose of living. The breakthrough you have during sports is physical, harmonious and a feeling of contentment. But on a so-called spiritual level it's more of a thankfulness which is very deep, very rewarding. It's again at a point where it's the feeling. When you're feeling the ecstasy of contentment and your mind says "this is heaven," you have probably dropped into your mind. It's on that level. It's not mind, it's serenity and gratitude. You have to fully live in the moment to experience that and then you will know. It will make you happy.

Character and Style

Character in skiing is when you look at a skier and can tell if they're aggressive or insecure. Are they relaxed and look like they're dancing? Are they tense and just want to race down the mountain like a thrill seeker? And if they are racing, are they careless of their surroundings are they putting themselves and the other skiers in danger? Because it is not about racing, it's about dancing. When you look at dancers, you can tell right away they're in harmony with the music. Yes, they have style and it's the same with skiing. Whether someone skis slow or fast you can tell if they're in control, if they're flowing or if they're in a bad mood and want to get their frustration out in skiing. Or they had too much to drink or smoked

The White Game

a joint, so instead of being clear or present they are experiencing the booze or the drug. If they are dancing and enjoying the skiing, they'll have much more joy instead of going down the hill like a crazy person where all they're feeling is frustration and fear that they're going to crash. This kind of skiing is dangerous.

When you're relaxed and flowing then you're much more aware of the condition of the day, for example, if it's a sunny day. Even when the conditions are difficult and you go at a cruising speed, then you're closer to harmony and that's when you become a beautiful skier. Let's call it style. Because style and harmony are related. When you look at that element you can see it in nature. You can feel it at the same time in your own experience of motion and your body. It's like hearing a symphony; you hear every note, you feel the motion and that's when you're truly dancing. That feeling of harmony can give you character because you can adapt that to everything you do in life. Whether you sit in an office or are driving a car being relaxed or being frustrated because of the traffic. Instead of being frustrated maybe you can get to a point that when you're alone you can sing to yourself; it's that simple.

Presence is also character forming. I've been skiing all

my life and that's why I am still crazy about it. When you see that experience in the details, in technique, and flowing through to breakthrough, it all becomes one. Instead of following your mind, you're at home; you're not doing anything. Visualize everything, and in your imagination you could be in the mountains dancing in the snow, and this vision relaxes you. When you open your eyes and you develop your awareness then you're surrounded by a lot of beauty. Vision leads to character. Vision, harmony, and character; they all come together.

Practicing vision will also teach you awareness and how it's all about being in the present moment, which will eventually give you a style not just of being a beautiful skier, but vice versa. People might say they're not a good skier yet they have beautiful style. This comes from being true to yourself and letting your experience come out because you've taken ideas and integrated them to let your true self manifest. You're confident and comfortable enough to express it in your own way. When you look at an instructor who has style, even if they ski slowly because they have some slow skiers, it looks totally natural and there is no retention of worry or anything negative. The client can be shaky and unsure, but the more they let go, the better they will look and that adds to their style and technique. We don't focus exclusively on technique, we talk about experience. You can relate to that state of being present because its character forming. We should experience that joy with everything we do and then it's much more pleasant. When you listen to a debate on TV where politicians deliberate over all these different ideas, and then they all agree on something, everybody is happy and relaxed. The other side of the debate is they are fighting, going through the motions and very often you see a lot of aggressiveness. There is so much antagonism, carelessness, and no style.

Style and the integration of these values are an expression of those important principles of feeling the moment called "now." Everything is connected. We're hooked up to every minute. The mind is the place where all the negative stuff is produced and since we don't practice much presence where the positive is, we open the door for aggressiveness and the dark stuff. That's why skiing is so wonderful. The snow and mountains are white, and white is connected to light, purity, and joy. It's part of the beauty of being relaxed and going at a certain pace. When we feel aggressiveness and tension as part of our day-to-day life, and we get up on the mountain, we don't even realize that by skiing down we will get rid

The Moment Called Now

of the frustration. It happens because we are in motion and in that there's a certain joy.

When you're present and you're on your way to go skiing or going to work then you feel good. You're looking forward to doing it, and doing it right. You're not stressed. When we have to rush and we're late then we don't enjoy it. Being conscious of our breathing in whatever we do has to become automatic because that's the source of our contentment. We do sports because they give us physical exercise, and when we're feeling it, then they give us a lot of energy. When we become conscious of that energy, we can also work out that's where the joy comes from. That's where the wellbeing comes from. When we're stressed and we have a lot on our plate, we easily get in the situation where if we would only just relax, the task would take just five minutes instead of hours. We don't manage to get it together because we have too many things on our mind.

When you're happy and content, you can feel it whether you are at work or are on your way to the office or going home. You can see when somebody is in that state. Even if they don't speak, their expression is contentment. To have that satisfaction, you have to practice being at peace with yourself. It's pleasant and we all know that

The White Game

because we like to enjoy life. But we've forgotten the feeling. It always comes back to that source. And practicing, it's that simple—to be or not to be.

Contentment speaks a different language. It's the language of the heart, of your true self. There is no bigger inspiration than to feel at peace, to be happy. That's what everybody aspires to and longs for. It's our most profound, most basic need. We must have it to become human again. I don't know if the world is going forward or backward. For the time being, we are really stuck. We have to clean up our act. We're trying everything and nothing works because we're ignoring the source of contentment. The magic is right there inside.

When someone has this quality of being content, we can call it style. Style is maybe not quite the word. It's more a form of happiness. It really comes to a point where all that is clarified when you practice presence and become conscious.

And if you can't find the feeling of presence, then ask for help. That's called thirst. The secret is to feel with the heart because that which we cannot put into words, where the heart is, is this huge mystery that is ultimately so simple. The heart opens when you feel the thirst for peace and when that happens it's beyond words. It's all there. Just stay in contact with that feeling by practicing presence. Because what is connecting you to your heart—it's your breath. That's it.

Personal Style

Living in the moment called "now" makes you content. And when you've mastered a sport through awareness, then it becomes pure enjoyment. You can do it until you can't walk anymore, and even then you can still talk about it. You know what it feels like and by talking about it you can feel a little bit of it without risking your neck. And it's good without the big boots, heavy skis, and clothes that make you feel like a fighting gladiator. You become very relaxed and that brings peace. Because you have mastered it, you can let go. You don't even care what it looks like.

You become free because when you have mastered something. You're not even proud of it. You're just thankful that you did all this skiing without getting hurt. And because you have done it you become a gratified skier. Now you can concentrate on another level to increase that nice feeling and go in a new direction. Instead of going out, you go in, and then you discover that there are infinite possibilities. But if you want to

The White Game

progress, you have to practice. The sincere desire to go deeper is enough to make you grow and give you the push. Maybe it's endless. Probably is.

If you think too much about your style, you will probably end up in your ego. And if you just do it for fun, then you enjoy it, and it doesn't matter. At that stage, you don't want to be the best or anything like that. It's just flowing and harmonious. At the end of the run, you feel content and you know that as far as style, it was good because you were totally relaxed. One with the snow, the sun, and the surroundings—just pure fun. You can't brag about it—you can only feel it. It's pure contentment, so there's not much you can say about it.

How do I describe the here and now without using a lot of words? It's a feeling of an experience that is harmonious. I have done it. I've mastered it. But the desire and hunger for more inner contentment and knowledge are still there. To sit down in the morning after washing my face with cold water and go inside is the most important thing for me. Instead of going outside where it's cold, and the equipment and ice and all the people are, I go inside where it's quiet and there is a fullness, peace, and tranquility which is beyond words.

We are using skiing as an example but it's actually about

our life and the quality of it. The more we concentrate on that quality and enjoy the feeling of presence, then our life will be filled with the good stuff. And the more we do it, the happier we will become. And in that respect, it's again about these three things: vision, character, and style.

Principles of Presence and the Flatland

Having a breakthrough is also possible off the mountain. For example, you walk on the beach and it's beautiful but the ocean has big waves, big breakers. You don't go swimming unless you're a really good swimmer. You respect nature. You can really enjoy just being there in safety and watching this floating element, which is part of us, and being still. That inner quiet we feel is the same force that drives these waves, the wind, and the clouds. Because you're watching that nature in safety it calms you down, gives you respect for the elements.

When you're driving a car, rushing around, and you're nervous and stressed, your movements become jerky. Then you can make the same thing happen—just slow down a little bit, breathe consciously and you'll be more relaxed. There's no situation where you can't calm yourself if you're conscious. It's always there because it's our life force. Might as well concentrate on it and use it. It's

The White Game

the gift that's given to us to help us because it gives us life. It really covers the whole scope of life—if we don't forget. It's there to help us. If you have a certain experience of this force, of this safe haven within you, then you start to flow. It becomes very pleasant, it relaxes you, it's healthy. The other stuff—when you look in the direction of hell—destroys you. And when you look to the source, you see the light.

The feeling of presence is everywhere, even if you're alone, not just in the mountains. When I worked as a steward on cruise ships during the off-season, after work I would go in the evening to a balcony at the back of the ship and just watch the movement of the boat on the ocean and it would feel good. It would calm me down and relax me. After a while, if I didn't have a jacket on and it got a little cool, I could go downstairs to my cabin, hit the bunk and I'd go into this heavenly sleep. The calming down functions the same way, whether it's in the mountains, an office, or the tropics. If you're conscious, the presence is always with you. Once it leaves you, forget it. It's gone. It's like a perfect safety belt. It can save you even when you don't know it, because you survive. With every breath something can happen and it just keeps going on. You get more into that side of living where there's harmony because in the mind is where everything dark lives too. And when you go there you get affected. If you stick to the other side then it's heavenly and if you're lucky, you know about the experience of gratitude. If you're not aware enough of it then you're a slave of the dark side. For us, the biggest gift is to know the right side and the power of it. It's like you can be in the middle of a hurricane and if you ask for help, it'll come.

Breath in the Here and Now

We can't stop our breath, it's always there, thank God. Conscious breathing is very important. It's essential for being able to relax, overcome fear, and recharge yourself. The more energy you have, the easier it is to let go. And when you get into the rhythm, there's no problem. Then you're breathing without concentrating, it's happening. The more you're relaxed, the more your breathing is in a rhythm too. You can practice it with whatever you do. If you're sitting in an office and you're stressed, what can you do? You stop and the first thing you do is take a really deep breath because you have to get that tension out. When you're conscious and take that breath, you very quickly re-energize. We all experience this at some point in our lives. We take this deep breath on and off, either because we lack energy or we're stressed or something like that, and then when we breathe deeply, the oxygen relaxes us.

Breathing properly has to be practiced. Whatever you do in this world or whatever work you do—maybe it's just sitting reading a book—you can very quickly find yourself lacking oxygen and then you have to breathe. That's why we take that big gulp and it should tell us that we should not just take one deep breath consciously but take four or five gulps of oxygen. You'll be more energized and relaxed and then you can go on working; if your job permits, take a little time out. That's the problem; every generation is stressed for one reason or another. However, breathe consciously and practice it; you'll be less stressed, if at all. You might even feel joy.

One Breath In

The role of the breath in being present is evident. When somebody has a bad tumble when skiing and finally stops and is OK, the first thing they do is take a deep breath and everything slows down. It makes you feel good, it gives you energy. You become calm. And when you're there again 100 percent, you can continue. We

The Moment Called Now

even take that breath without knowing—it's spontaneous. If the body has tension, it'll take that breath. You're a little stressed and then you feel the tension go away when the body sighs. That's already enough to put you back into balance mentally and physically.

The body will do it when it needs to. You don't have to be conscious of it. That's why all of a sudden, we experience there is this inhale and we take that breath. If the stress isn't too big, we've already slowed down and become present again. We can feel again. When we're in stress and the body needs to slow down, we're totally out of harmony. Then when that energy comes in with the breath—it's like an instant tranquilizer. It's natural, you don't even have to take a pill. People could also use relaxed deep breathing when they have certain pains or something like that. They don't necessarily always have to take medicine. You can learn to slow yourself down and let go and then the tension loosens up and you're OK. That's the gift. At the same time, it's proof of the miracle that I'm still alive. Breathing—it's our life stream.

Through our modern way of living, we actually give breath very little or no importance. We never think about it. We just concentrate on making more money and get more aggressive. It creates this short circuit in the system. You start getting uptight and hostile so you need to slow down again. And that's conscious breathing—letting go—let the body breathe. Not in a certain way—let it do its thing. We often say "control your breathing." You can't really control it because it knows itself what to do. It can do it best because it's coming from a source, which is the source of everything. It knows best when to give life to this freaked out creature. If you let it be in charge, then we're in harmony—there's no problem. The problems can't even come close except if a rock hits us on our head when we're on a mountain. Breathing should really be conscious breathing, and integrated in our culture. Not for a spiritual reason, just for moment-to-moment living, day to day, because that's where it all comes from.

The Journey is the Destination

When you're happy and content then you're on the journey of life. You want to be on that journey all the time because it is complete, it has both the finite and infinite. How can you describe it when there is no end and no beginning of that enjoyment? It was always there and it always will be. I can only say practice presence because you will enjoy it more and more.

The Moment Called Now

When I was a skier I used to have the reputation that I was the loveliest skier and I didn't have to win any races. When I skied I felt like I was flying. After I had a good run in deep powder I would stop and have the feeling I was overflowing in this fulfillment. That's our basic need, we always want more of this feeling. And you can always have more. It's like a breakthrough in life, that's what it is. Practice it and you will be more fully alive in the present moment. We've been talking about a breakthrough in skiing but the real breakthrough is knowing how to be present.

When you practice presence, it becomes a basic need. You need that contentment. You need that happiness. You need to be with people who understand that kind of language. It becomes the basic need of feeling the contact with that energy that is beating your heart. You can hear the pulse like a clock when you are quiet. That's your true clock. It started when you were born; when you took your first breath. You'll be with it to the end of your days. It's the energy that's driving all this, always was, and always will be. Once you reach that joy of feeling presence then you get addicted. Divine addiction. Perfect. It has no judgment anymore. That negative side of the world disappears and it becomes pure.

The White Game

The White Game is this beautiful experience of the snow. It has a very magic side to it. When it falls and snows very heavily you can start to hear it. It's like a drizzling. When it snows and it becomes night and keeps snowing you go to sleep and when you wake up the weather is clear. The sun is coming out and there's fresh snow with billions of little lights blinking on the surface. Even though there are billions of flakes and no two are alike, they're all lighting up. The light has a magic consistency and it looks like it's very alive and very miraculous. When you go up on a lift or a gondola and you see this blinking of the first snow because the sun is out and the snow is reflecting it, it's like being alive. It's total magic. Be still and just watch the magic. That's why I call it The White Game.

The White Game has a big aspect. From within, from without. From within you see it much better. You even get to the point where you see it and experience the miracle. It's a beautiful part of creation. It's what we want to know about because it's so beautiful. It feels magical when you glide into it. You come to the point where you become euphoric. It's where you can try and describe it but the only real thing you can do is to experience it.

The Moment Called Now

One part is just the idea because we have a certain experience, but when we really let go we see the magic. That's what gives us that joy. That fulfilling feeling of being one with an aspect of creation. You play the real game.

These are a lot of beautiful words but it's only the shadow of what we experience. I hope this isn't sounding too mystical because it's not. It's real, it's totally real. Even talking about it, it becomes real. I know it's true because I've experienced it. I have to believe it. It's true in the truest sense. Presence gives you an understanding and an appreciation that you literally feel. You feel that harmony so that it's almost like the breakthrough. The breakthrough is at a very harmonious slow pace like in a gentle movement or even at high speed. It's not in the limited space of the action. It has no borders. When you break through in skiing and stop, you have that vision of light sparkling and being fulfilled. You can describe it, but only by feeling and living it can you understand what it is. Then it also becomes free of ego because it feels like gratitude. It's such an incredible feeling I almost don't dare to speak of it because it's more than words.

I would call it becoming joyful instead of aggressive. When you consciously see the two, you have no problem choosing the right thing. You just go for it. But don't

The White Game

forget you need to have the thirst. When your heart hears that and there is sincerity, then it will open. Then you let go and it will manifest. That's when the dance starts. And if you keep it going, it will never end. Never.

It holds everything you ever wanted. It doesn't matter anymore where you are, what you do, what you have, or what you don't have. You know the secret. By practicing presence, you also have this magic clarity where whatever you see, hear, or feel is this divine energy. You become aware of that omnipresence.

What would the world be like if presence was a way of life for everybody? It would be paradise. I don't want to pretend I'm always in paradise, I'm still at the beginning but that's what's so fantastic. It's getting better and better. Even though I'm getting older, it doesn't diminish the contentment or my happiness and my enthusiasm. Because everything grows: your clarity, your understanding. It's all part of our basic need to be happy. I think we're all looking for something and it will become clear by itself from experiencing what's happening all around us. Just enjoy it and then the universe will do the rest. Maybe the universe wants us to dance a little longer, celebrate, and we do.

Acknowledgments

There are many people and organizations who have supported me over the years of my skiing life that I wish to thank. I will start by thanking my father who first put me on skis and supported my early days with his patience and wisdom. I am forever grateful to The Swiss National Ski Team for selecting me to represent Switzerland. It was an honor and source of many good memories. The Swiss Ski School Zermatt were most generous for giving me my start as a teacher and later providing many wonderful clients when I became independent. The musical entrepreneur extraordinaire Claude Nobbs, an inspired student and friend who recommended me to the musicians visiting his Montreux Jazz Festivals for which I am very appreciative. The ski life would not have been as much fun without the most incredible après ski activities the Ivarsson family hosted for the countless memorable nights at the Hotel Post. Many thanks to Tim Gallwey who has been a good friend for many years and shared with me numerous insights from the Inner Game that inspired my own teaching. A special thanks to Christine Gentinetta for always being there for me and being the perfect partner.

---- Peter Kronig

There are many people who helped make this book accessible both textually and visually that I would like to thank. Anne Gillion for excellent editing and word-smithing to help to make the text flow. Roz Morris for providing structural insights and editorial review. Helen Baggott for precise proofreading and perfecting the language. Anna Taylor at Taylormade GmbH for her inspiring cover design and graphic support that made the book come alive. Lin White for her expert layout that makes the book ultimately both readable and pleasurable for the eyes. Especially grateful to the early readers Kathy Miller, Typhaine Le Corvec and Lara Affuso who shared feedback to help the project along and Tanya Greiner, Rani Thoms, Elisabeth Fransdonk, John MacArthur and Andrina Tisi who helped find the best title possible.

---- Chris Corbett

Acknowledgments

Both of us wish to thank Prem Rawat who originally suggested to write a book about this teaching approach when he and his family were Peter's ski students. We're especially grateful for his friendship, inspiration, support and reminding us to always find the joy in the moment called now.

Peter Kronig has been skiing since he was three years old. He joined the Swiss National Ski team as a downhill and slalom racer when he was a teenager and certified as a teacher in the Swiss Ski School. In his early twenties when he wasn't teaching, he worked as a photo model in Paris and New York, spending time with top designers from St. Laurent to Halston.

He has taught students all around the world – USA, Canada, France, Switzerland and South America - all with very effective results. Because of his high standard of teaching he's been able to work with an elite clientele that includes private bankers, business executives, politicians, doctors, rock stars, Academy Award winning film directors and European royalty.

From the very beginning of his career he has worked with private clients and gradually refined the techniques and insights that were based on his natural style of teaching.

Being a meditation practitioner since the 1970's he has been able to combine insights from his studies with practical exercises to successfully increase human potential.

Chris Corbett is the author of the novel Nirvana Blues. He was born in the UK with the creative background of a grandfather who was a best-selling author in 1920's London as well as the first Artistic Director of the BBC.

He grew up in Northern California where he was educated at the University of California in Berkeley and Santa Cruz while also studying yoga and meditation. Moving to Los Angeles he worked for Playboy Magazine, Walt Disney and on an Academy Award winning film in addition to documentary film projects in Europe, America and India. He also owned a publishing business for eight years, operating from one of the oldest film studios in Hollywood.

Since moving to Zurich, Switzerland he has been working as a corporate communications professional at the global headquarters of several international companies. He is a regular contributor to the Huffington Post, Medium and Thrive, had his fiction work published in a short story collection and is currently working on a second novel.